Apple Cider Vinegar

Other Books by Victoria Rose

Fiction

Cloud Hidden, Whereabouts Unknown
Christina—A Sci/Fi Fantasy Romance
Toni—A Sci/Fi Fantasy Romance
Josy—A Sci/Fi Fantasy Romance
The Rose Sisters Trilogy
Trust Me, the Devil Said

Nonfiction

Ladies, Are You Lost?—
Options for Women in Unhealthy Relationships

Apple Cider Vinegar

History and Folklore—Composition—Medical Research
—Medicinal, Cosmetic, and Household Uses—
Commercial and Home Production

Victoria Rose
Author of Ladies, Are You Lost?

iUniverse, Inc.
New York Lincoln Shanghai

Apple Cider Vinegar
History and Folklore—Composition—Medical Research—Medicinal,
Cosmetic, and Household Uses—Commercial and Home Production

Copyright © 2006 by Helena Gunther

iUniverse books may be ordered through booksellers or by contacting:

iUniverse
2021 Pine Lake Road, Suite 100
Lincoln, NE 68512
www.iuniverse.com
1-800-Authors (1-800-288-4677)

ISBN-13: 978-0-595-41237-2 (pbk)
ISBN-13: 978-0-595-85591-9 (ebk)
ISBN-10: 0-595-41237-8 (pbk)
ISBN-10: 0-595-85591-1 (ebk)

Printed in the United States of America

This book is dedicated to Ross Johnson who left planet Earth August 17, 2006, for a new adventure. Thank you for calling to say good-bye. You live in my heart and mind, and I will always love you.

CONTENTS

INTRODUCTION

Greetings, oh gentle reader, and welcome to the written world of apple cider vinegar. As you are now reading this introduction, I might imagine that you have some interest in taking responsibility for your own health and well-being; perhaps cider vinegar folk remedies enchant you; you're looking for a new hobby; you liked the color or design of my book cover; or, like myself, the word "why" has been a part of your vocabulary since you began to talk. Whatever your reasons, welcome!

With so many books and magazines available today on just about every subject, why write another book and why a book about apple cider vinegar (ACV)? Because: **This book answers questions about apple cider vinegar that have not been asked before**. There are other books on cider vinegar; some are listed in my bibliography. One book focuses on vinegars in general. Another book focuses on the health benefits of cider vinegar but claims there are no cider vinegars on the market of any nutritional value, yet provides no information where to find good cider vinegar or how to make it. This book gives you information about market brands and how to make your own.

An awareness has been growing in the holistic health field of the natural therapeutic value and dynamic versatility of apple cider vinegar. The therapeutic and medicinal value is supported by medical and scientific research. **This book will provide you with medical evidence to support why apple cider vinegar works for so many common ailments.**

As you grow to have more confidence in this natural product of Nature, you will want more information about the brands currently on the market, particularly if you plan to add ACV to your regular health program. There are many questions to be asked about the quality of available brands. Are organic apples used? Are waxed peels included in the pressing of the juice? Are raw, unfiltered cider vinegars better? What are the truths about additives and pasteurization? Is apple cider vinegar made from apples today? **This book will help you find the answer to many questions about the quality of cider vinegar available today.**

After reading the information provided here on some of the brands currently on the market and after researching and experimenting on your own with market brands, you might possibly want to consider making your own cider vinegar. Making your own will give you control over the selection of the variety of apples used, the blend, the quality of apples (organic and non-waxed), and it will be your choice whether or not to include peels and cores. You will have choices: additives or not, pasteurization or not. One thing you have going for you when you make your own is *time*. By letting your cider vinegar age and mature, much of the sediments will settle out, eliminating the need for additives. Commercial producers today do not have the time or storage space for aging and maturing because of the volume they process. They use additives to speed up the clarification process. If you think you are ready for a new healthful hobby, the product of which will make caring gifts for friends and family (along with a copy of the book), **this book will provide you with step-by-step directions for making your own ACV—from setting up your own work space, pressing your apples, to bottling and labeling your end product.**

I have not included in this book personal case histories to demonstrate or substantiate the medicinal benefits of ACV. I prefer to use information or documented research as support because there is no control factor in personal case histories. What worked for Aunt Sue might not work for Uncle Joe. Who knows what Aunt Sue was doing or taking when the remedy worked for her.

I have tried to present the material in this book on three levels:

1. The first level is directed to readers who just want to use the book as a reference for cider vinegar uses and to possibly make their own;

2. The second level includes the first but also provides a broader perspective on the subject to readers interested in the history and medical research; and

3. The third includes the first and second and then provides the technical and scientific information necessary for readers who need specifics.

If you find the history and technical data not to your taste, just move on. It may be of interest to you another day. **The core of this book is the dynamic versatility of apple cider vinegar.**

CHAPTER 1

HISTORY OF VINEGARS

Vinegar and cider are included in this history because they are related, and there is more evidence of their use down through recorded history. Vinegar is one of the oldest fermentation products known to man. The oldest is wine, from which the first vinegar was made. Cider is the fermented alcoholic drink from apple juice. Cider vinegar is the fermented vinegar from alcoholic cider.

Intoxicating drinks have been around almost as long as man. Wines were made from fruits, vegetables and grains. The early people did not understand the fermentation processes, but they did understand the effects of the end products–alcohol and vinegar. Generally, what they did not understand, they attributed to an act of God or a favor from some spirit deity. Wines were included in religious ceremonies. When the wine or alcoholic drink went sour, it had fermented into vinegar and was then used for drink, preserving and medicinal purposes.

EARLY HISTORY

As early as 5000 B.C. the Babylonians made wine from date palm, and the Egyptians made wine from barley.

The Aryans, a nomadic tribe that roamed Northern Europe and Asia, first appeared in history around 2500 B.C. These Aryans, or Indo-Europeans–ancestors of India, Greece, Italy and all Germanic, Celtic, Anglo-Saxon, Scandinavian and Slavic peoples–developed a taste for "soured apple wine," the forerunner of apple cider. The name "cider" is rooted in the Phoenician "shekar," meaning wine or strong drink. From the Babylonians and Aryans, to the Phoenicians, "soured wine" passed on to the Greek and Roman empires.

Discorides, in his travels with Nero's army through Egypt, documented the use of vinegar for medicinal purposes. Vinegar alone or combined with honey was used for a variety of illnesses. Egyptians used it for mushroom poisoning, loss of appetite, ear problems, wounds and gangrene (Diggs 1989).

Hippocrates used vinegar as a medicine. He recommended a drink called oxymel, which was a combination of vinegar and honey, for expectoration, freedom of breathing, constipation, fever, peri-pneumonia and pleuritic affections.

The Romans purified their drinking water by adding wine vinegar. Pliny, a well-known naturalist, noted in his writings that Cleopatra once dissolved pearls in vinegar to win a bet with Mark Anthony that she would consume at a single meal the value of a million sesterces (an ancient Roman coin of considerable monetary value). He also wrote of the excellent quality of vinegar made from Cyprus figs and Alexandria figs. Around 77 A.D. he wrote of a natural juice from apples.

Julius Caesar led two Roman legions to England in 55 B.C. and discovered cider to be the common drink. The apple was a sacred fruit to the Celtics according to their mythology, and an apple god was worshiped by many early tribes in England.

Titus Livius chronicling Hannibal's march to Rome, reported that the soldiers set fire to wood placed at the base of large rocks in their path and then poured vinegar on the hot rocks to crack them. They then chiseled through the softened boulders.

Jewish people drank a mixture of vinegar and water daily. They were forbidden to drink this mixture on the Day of Atonement because of its relaxing effect. They used vinegar in various recipes, to wet the flat loaves of bread they ate, for smoothing and cooling the body, as an astringent, for toothaches, as a gargle and for wounds and dandruff.

Vinegar is mentioned in the Bible. The Book of Ruth, 2nd Chapter, 14th Verse: "And Boza said unto her, 'At meal time come hither, and eat of the bread, and dip thy morsel in the vinegar....'" The Book of Numbers makes reference to drinking vinegar. It was a common practice to dip pieces of bread into vinegar.

There are records in China of vinegar being used as a food preservative in the Zhou, Han and Qin periods. Vinegar was a staple of the Chinese diet during the Tang and Chen dynasties. Crab applies, pears, plums, raw walnuts, onions, meat and fish were put up and preserved with vinegar to be used for special, festive occasions.

The Japanese learned rice wine- and vinegar-making techniques from China. The written records of the uses of vinegar in Japan are in the Imperial Archives (Diggs 1989).

Cider was known and consumed in much of Europe in the 3rd century. In France, Charlemagne enforced laws to promote and control the manufacture and production of cider. A French authority, G. Warcollier, claimed that cider was more popular than beer in the 11th and 12th centuries. In England hard cider was a popular rural drink up to the 12th century. It was as potent as most beers and cheaper. Every farmer made cider for his family and help. The land gentry owned large presses to furnish tenants with cider.

Vinegar–from the French vinaigre, vin for wine and aigre meaning sour–continued to be a by-product of wine making until 1670 when the French began to commercially process vinegar in Orleans. Vinegar gave the French cuisine its unequaled "cooking with wine" reputation.

18TH AND 19TH CENTURIES

In England around the 18th century about two thousand varieties of apples were grown. Many scientific methods had been developed to improve and speed up the production of cider. Treatises began to appear on making cider. A Dutch technologist, Hermann Boerhaave, found that the rate of acid production in the vinegar process was directly proportional to the amount of surface exposed to air. Thus, subsequent methods attempted to introduce more air into the casks. A French doctor/scientist, Dr. Edouard Denis-Dumont born in 1830, spent his life researching the natural therapeutic value of cider. In 1865 the French physicist Louis Pasteur showed that it is the bacteria in vinegar that cause the conversion of alcohol to acetic acid. A group of organisms work together symbiotically, producing enough acid to prevent invasion by other organisms. A number of these agents have been isolated under the genus name Acetobacter (Orton 1973).

AMERICAN HISTORY

Apples and cider are a part of American history. Cider apples, however, were not indigenous to the North American continent. There is no evidence that the Native Americans used crab apples to make cider. The English brought apple seeds with them. John Chapman, also known as Johnny Appleseed, brought the first apples and apple cider to the Alleghenies. Apple trees were planted in the Massachusetts Bay Colony. Historical records reveal that cider was an integral part of everyday life of rural folk in 19th century New England. Cider presses were a part of the New England landscape. Cider was drunk in homes, inns and taverns. It was a part of daily life and served at gatherings, from house and barn raising to military functions. The consumption of cider in the 19th century reached such a high level that in 1874 the National Women's Christian Temperance Union was formed to limit or stop its use, but consumption continued to rise.

The second president of the United States, John Adams, drank a tankard of hard cider every morning before breakfast and lived to be ninety one. During the campaign for President in 1840, the Whigs nominated General William Harrison for President and John Tyler for Vice President. To emphasize Harrison's humble origin, the prime campaign symbol was a barrel of cider. The campaign headquarters was located in a log cabin. A barrel of cider sat outside in front of the cabin. Cider was served free to all who could vote. General Harrison won the Presidency by an electoral landslide.

In the United States the Heinz Company has been producing vinegar since 1880 and was the first food firm to market vinegars in individual glass bottles for the consumer.

CHAPTER 2

WHAT IS APPLE CIDER VINEGAR?

Robert L. La Belle, Professor of Food Science at Cornell's State Agriculture Experiment Station at Geneva, New York, stated in his 1971 monograph:

"In my opinion...the term fresh, sweet or farm cider should be reserved for the simple old-fashioned product, normally oxidized in color and flavor and still containing all the suspended solids that render it almost opaque.... However, all processing, such as heating or the addition of ascorbic acid that largely prevents oxidation, produces 'apple juice,' not cider."

Richard H. Case, writing for the Herald American, quoted a New York farmer as saying, "The only way to have real cider is just as it comes from the press. When you start putting things in to preserve it, you spoil the flavor."

DEFINITION

Cider vinegar is defined as a vinegar made from the juice of apples which has passed through two fermentation processes–alcoholic and acetification. The sugar in the apple juice is first converted to alcohol by yeast of the genus Saccharomyces. Acetic acid bacteria (Acetobacter) transform the alcohol into acetic acid.

There is an imitation, cider-flavored vinegar on the market made from coal tar. It looks pure and tastes like vinegar. Synthetic vinegar made by diluting concentrated (glacial) acetic acid with water is also available. Distilled vinegar, also known as grain, spirit or white vinegar, is made from industrial alcohol and used primarily as a preservative. Malt vinegar, very popular in England, is made from barley and oats.

The first legal definition of vinegar in the United States was defined by the Federal Food and Drugs Act of 1906. In 1933 it was revised and six types of vinegar were defined. Under those guidelines the unqualified term 'vinegar' could only be used to designate apple cider vinegar.

BASIC PRODUCTION PHASES

An apple orchard in full, spring-time bloom is a marvelous sight. The fragrance is heavenly. Busy bees work in the warm sun to collect nectar and pollinate the blossoms so an apple will be produced. Man's work begins in the autumn and peaks in October and November. The ripe apples are gathered into trucks and trailers for delivery to factories. The apples are graded upon arrival and then put into silos. They are washed, moved into the pressing house, passed through a rotary drum for a final wash and reduced to pulp. A press squeezes all the juice out. The juice rests in vats to settle before being pumped into storage vats for fermentation into alcohol. This fermentation starts at once and is caused by the action of natural yeasts which are in the air and present on the outer skin of apples. Fermentation continues until the sugar in the juice has been converted to alcohol and carbonic acid gas. The conversion of sugars to alcohol by yeast is well understood. This process generally takes about three to four weeks.

The next process will be making cider vinegar. The alcoholic and acetous fermentation processes are completely separate operations. Acetification is the final process. The conversion of alcohol to acetic acid is less well understood. The traditional process was to acetify in vats of Columbian pine or New Zealand Kauri pine, but stainless steel, fibre glass and glass-lined steel vats are used today.

Despite its ancient origin, the technology of vinegar production advanced slowly, improvements consisting principally of better methods of aeration. The more oxygen you can get to the bacteria, the faster the cider will process into acetic acid. There are three basic methods used to produce vinegar. The slow process, the generator process and the submerged process. The Orleans or French process is the best known of the old methods. Acetification is done by the Acetobacter bacteria. This bacteria converts the alcohol into acetic acid. When the acetification process is over, the cider vinegar is filtered and stored to develop flavor and remove sediment.

If the right nutritive conditions are maintained, the bacteria produce enzymes which cause the oxidation of the alcohol. These nutrients include simple sugars (glucose), amino acids and other nitrogenous compounds, vitamins, particularly of the B complex and inorganic compounds, especially phosphates. The chemical reaction is most simply represented as:

$$CH_3CH_2OH + O_2 + bacterial\ enzymer = CH_3COOH + H_2O.$$

Problems arise as producers need to speed up the process because of increased volume, lack of storage space and the customer's desire for a clear, bright product. This will be discussed in the section on Commercial Production.

COMPOSITION

Apple cider vinegar will vary in composition depending upon the type of apples used. The major component of cider vinegar, apart from water, is acetic acid. Any table of values compiled from various sources should be used only as a guide to the composition of cider vinegars. The following is a basic breakdown of composition: Total solid matter, acetic acid, sugars, mineral ash, tannin, protein, calcium phosphorus, potassium, sodium, iron, lead, arsenic, copper, zinc, riboflavin, nicotinic acid, ascorbic acid (Bragg 1989).

Fraud in cider vinegars may sometimes be detected by the presence of mineral acid or sulfate, by the absence of amino acids and by the absence of B vitamins. Carbon isotope ratios can distinguish between "natural" acetic acid produced by fermentation and "chemical" acetic acid synthesized from petroleum products. Fermentation of petroleum-derived ethanol will produce acetic acid with a carbon isotope ratio characteristic of the synthetic product. In the "Vagabond Vinegar" case, the FDA in San Juan, Puerto Rico, required that a producer of acetic acid correct their labeling to include the word "Imitation" immediately preceding the word "vinegar" on the label (FDA Consumer 1988).

Cider vinegars may be distinguised from other vinegars by their relatively high content or sorbitol, and possibly by the presence of unique phenolic compounds such as phloridzin, which are detectable chromatographically. The absence of malic acid is no proof that a vinegar is not derived from cider, since the action of lactic acid bacteria during the initial cider making or storage can convert all the malic acid to lactic acid. Both malic and lactic acid may have disappeared by the end of acetification.

Kahn et al. (1972) reported that the major volatile constituents of cider vinegars other than acetic acid were acetaldehyde, ethyl formate, ethyl acetate, ethanol, isobutanol, 2-methylbutanol, isopentanol and 2-phenyl ethanol. Other carbonyls, esters and alcohols were also detected. The volatile distribution changes with the different acetification processes.

SPECIFICATIONS

The analytical specifications for cider vinegar are basically simple. Limits are set for the following characteristics: (1) total acidity; (2) alcohol; (3) iron, copper and heavy metal content; (4) appearance or turbidity; and (5) color.

The values as established by the Vinegar Institute in the United States are listed in the following table. The test method is given in *Official Methods of Analysis*, 12th ed., 1975, published by the Association of Official, Analytical Chemists, Washington, DC.

Table 1—Specification for Cider Vinegar

Characteristic	Limit
Acid content.........	4.0 g/100ml minimum, expressed as acetic acid
Appearance..........	Clear, bright liquid
Color.................	Light to medium amber satisfactory to consumer and producer
Odor.................	Clean, fruity satisfactory to consumer and producer
Trace metals	
Copper............	5.0 ppm maximum
Iron................	10.0 ppm maximum
Heavy Metals......	1.0 ppm maximum
Alcohol content......	0.5% by volume maximum

Credit: Vinegar Institute (1978)

In addition, the Vinegar Institute requires the following: "Cider vinegar shall be made by the alcoholic and subsequent acetous fermentation of the juice of apples or concentrate thereof. Each shipment is guaranteed, as of the date of delivery, not to be adulterated nor misbranded within the meaning of the Federal Food, Drug and Cosmetic Act. Product shall be manufactured in accordance with the Federal guidelines for Good Manufacturing Practices."

Any additives such as sulfur dioxide or ascorbic acid must be monitored. Turbidity will often times be assessed by eye. A spectrophotometer can be used. An initial turbidity of less than 10 NTU is required by basic specifications. A reference sample may be used for visual color comparison to meet color specifications.

CHAPTER 3

MEDICAL RESEARCH RELATING TO CIDER VINEGAR

The documentation of the effectiveness of cider vinegar as a medicinal aid starts with its history. Hippocrates recommended a drink called oxymel, a combination of vinegar and honey, for promoting expectoration to help breathing and for other lung related conditions.

Dr. Edouard Denis-Dumont, born 1830, spent his life researching the natural therapeutic value of cider and performing clinical experiments using cider for medicinal purposes. His treatise on the relation of cider to the incidence of gallbladder disease, kidney stones, gout, diabetes, dental and urinary problems can be considered the first major study of cider by a trained scientist.

Physicians have recommended cider vinegar for various ailments throughout history. Studies have shown that cider

14

vinegar is extremely valuable in the body's biochemical operations. Vinegar is an essential building block in the construction of many complex substances in the body.

ACETIC ACID

A number of studies were carried out at four different universities. One study tagged atoms to trace the path of cider vinegar through the tissues and cells. This allowed the students to see how the body used the vinegar.

Acetic acid, the principal constituent in vinegar, plays an important role in the release of energy from fats and carbohydrates. Cider vinegar helps in the processing of fats, glucose, amino acids and hemoglobin. Dr. Konrad F. Block of Columbia University said that acetic acid is carried by the blood into the kidneys and muscles and undergoes complete oxidation with the release of energy. Some of the cider vinegar is retained and utilized as a source of carbon atoms for the synthesis of a variety of tissue constituents.

Dr. F. Lipman of Massachusetts General Hospital has done research to prove that acetic acid aids in detoxifying the body from drugs which have been taken by making them more easily excreted.

Dr. Irving L. Ochs of Annapolis, Maryland, has done research which demonstrated that acetic acid acts as a bactericidal agent. He used cider vinegar to treat external Otitis, a severe form of ear infection. In his treatment of the Otitis, he first cleaned the ear with hydrogen peroxide and then put in the ear a piece of cotton saturated with 5 percent strength cider vinegar. He continued this treatment for up to a week, checking daily for reduction in pain and swelling. The skin returned to normal in about a week. This treatment is used today for diseases caused by Pseudomonas, Candida and Aspergillus (Diggs 1989).

Research has proven that a 5 percent concentration of acetic acid is lethal to many microorganisms. Lower concentrations have been found to be quite effective. A 1 percent solution is used prophylactically in surgical dressings, and a .25 percent solution is used in catheterization and irrigation of the bladder. Vaginal infections caused by Candida and Trichomonas are treated with douche solutions of .25 percent to 1 percent. These solutions are also used as a spermatocide. Concentrations of 5 percent have been found to be effective in treating extensive burns. Dr. C. R. Owen also demonstrated the bactericidal properties of acetic acid against gram-negative bacteria (Diggs 1989).

ACID-ALKALINE BALANCE

Acid-alkaline balance is necessary for normal functioning of cells in the body. Through intricate body mechanisms the various acids and alkalines which enter the blood stream are neutralized or eliminated. This keeps the blood's acid-alkaline ratio constant. This balance is evaluated on a scale of 10 to 14 with 7 being neutral. Seven to 14 is an alkaline reaction. A factor of 1 is equal to 100 times increase in pH. This means that acid is 100 times stronger at 5 than at 6.

Until recently most doctors agreed that the normal pH or acid-alkaline balance was alkaline. Now, newer evidence reveals that an acid pH in the stomach and urine and a slightly alkaline pH in the blood are ideal for optimum health and body functioning. During the flushing and cleansing of the body, the pH is alkaline, but it definitely needs to be acid for healing to take place (Malstrom 1977).

It is very easy to test your own urine in the morning when you get up. You can purchase testing paper either at your pharmacy or local health food store. Testing your urine will give you some indication as to the acid-alkaline balance of your system.

If you find that your urine is exceptionally alkaline, apple cider vinegar can help to restore the balance so that the urine will test more acid in reaction. Start with a tablespoon of cider vinegar in an eight ounce glass of water. Drink this mixture before breakfast and with each meal until your urine test shows an acid reaction.

Your skin also is healthier with an acid mantle. If you have dry, flaky, itchy skin, your system is most likely too alkaline. A cider vinegar bath with about two cups of vinegar will help restore this acid mantle. Along with helping the skin, this bath will also help sore, tired muscles and relax you in general.

HYDROCHLORIC ACID AND DIGESTION

The human digestive system consists of the alimentary canal, extending from the mouth to the rectum. Accessory organs supply necessary enzymes and substances to aid digestion. The tongue, teeth, salivary glands, pancreas, liver and gall bladder are these accessory organs.

Insufficient amounts of hydrochloric acid in the stomach will result in symptoms of indigestion due to delay in the emptying time of the stomach, indigestion of protein and non-destruction of acid-fast bacteria. Foods putrefy in the stomach which causes gas, bloating and discomfort. Hydrochloric acid is very essential for the systemic assimilation of calcium and other minerals.

The person with complete absence of hydrochloric acid is most likely a very sick person. When the stomach empties very slowly, little or no food is digested or assimilated. Lactic acid, a forerunner to cancer, is formed.

Conditions and problems such as anemia, arthritis, colitis and tourista-diarrhea can be prevented with proper amounts of hydrochloric acid during digestion.

Symptoms of Hydrochloric Acid Deficiency

To determine if there is a deficiency in hydrochloric acid, watch for fruit juice souring in the stomach, gas and bloating after each meal, halitosis, poor digestion and poor assimilation of food.

Supplements to Correct Hydrochloric Acid Deficiency

Apple cider vinegar blended with honey is a recommended source to build up hydrochloric acid. Kelp and azomite are also natural sources to build up this acid. Tablets of hydrochloric acid combined with betain and pepsin are also a good supplemental source. Care should be taken when using the hydrochloric acid tablets not to take too much, and they must be taken with a meal. A raw vegetable diet is recommended as an acidifier. Vinegar baths and enemas are also suggested to correct this deficiency.

If there is any pain or adverse reaction to a cider vinegar drink, discontinue using the drink as this may indicate an ulcer or that your system is too acidic. See your physician (Malstrom 1977).

Commercial antacids in any form, including bicarbonate of soda, increase the deficiency of hydrochloric acid and ultimately add to digestive problems.

POTASSIUM

Dr. DeForest C. Jarvis, a graduate of the College of Medicine at the University of Vermont, practiced Ophthalmology and Otolaryngology in Barre, Vermont, in 1909. His interest in the natural properties of apple cider vinegar was a hobby he pursued throughout his life. He did extensive research in Vermont with the help of the local people. His theories are based on studies of old folk remedies.

His book, *Folk Medicine: A Vermont Doctor's Guide to Good Health*, is a classic in scientific research on the medicinal properties of cider vinegar. The book goes into great detail about his studies with animals and humans. The applications of old folk remedies were applied to cure human ills, to prevent sickness and to maintain good health by natural means. His theory was applied to the treatment of many problems, i.e. arthritis, kidney trouble, obesity, hypertension, fatigue, headaches, etc. One of the therapeutic remedies made popular by Dr. Jarvis was a mixture of natural strained honey and natural cider vinegar. There is an extensive record of significant clinical data to support his studies.

His focus centered on the potassium found in cider vinegar. He saw humans and animals go to great length to get the potassium that their bodies wanted. There would be no life if there was no potassium. It is one of the most widely distributed tissue minerals but never occurs in a free state. It is always combined with an acid.

In the garden, potassium is necessary for the production of the substances which give rigidity to the plant stems. It increases the plant's resistance to disease. Potassium deficiency in a plant is indicated by a cessation of growth for no apparent reason. If the deficiency is not corrected, the plan will slowly yellow and die. Similarly in the human body, when we notice the presence of abnormal growth or failure to replace worn-out tissues, this could be indicative of insufficient potassium. Uncontrolled growth might be a tendency to callous formations on the soles of the feet. Failure to replace worn-out tissues might be observed in loss of hair, decayed teeth and fingernails that bend and tear.

Functions of Potassium

Without potassium your heart would not beat and nerve signals would not be transmitted. It is to the soft tissues what calcium is to the hard tissues of the body. It slows up the hardening processes that menace the whole blood-vessel system. It softens arteries and keeps them flexible and resilient. It is the mineral of youthfulness, and it fights bacteria and viruses. Bacteria need moisture to maintain themselves and get it by taking moisture from body cells. If there is enough potassium in each body cell, the potassium will draw moisture from the bacteria instead.

Potassium is one of the electrolytes, mineral salts that conduct electricity when dissolved in water. Electrolytes are always found in pairs. A positive molecule, such as sodium or potassium, is always accompanied by a negative molecule, such as chloride. As a major electrolyte, potassium is involved in maintaining normal water balance and distribution, acid-alkaline balance, muscle and nerve cell functions, heart functions, kidney and adrenal functions. It is also essential for the conversion of blood sugar into glycogen, the stored form of blood sugar found in the muscles and liver.

Symptoms of Potassium Deficiency

When there is a potassium deficiency, there is a slow degeneration of body cells and premature aging. This deficiency affects muscles and nerves first. Less glycogen is being stored and because glycogen is used by muscles for energy, a potassium deficiency will produce great fatigue and muscle weakness. These are some of the first signs of this deficiency.

Mental confusion, irritability, heart disturbances, lower back aches and pains, morning headaches, dull hair, itchy scalp, premature balding, itchy eyes, bloodshot and watery eyes, forgetfulness and memory failure, difficulty in making decisions are also signs of a potassium deficiency.

Dietary potassium deficiency is more common in the elderly and is generally caused by a diet low in fresh fruit and vegetables and high in sodium. It is more common that a deficiency is due to excessive fluid loss caused by sweating, diarrhea or urination and by the use of diuretics, laxatives, aspirin and other drugs. The amount of potassium lost in sweat can be quite significant, especially if the exercise is prolonged in a warm climate (Senior Counselor 1991).

A shortage of potassium can cause a potentially fatal condition known as hypokalemia, typically resulting from diarrhea, increased diuresis and vomiting. Symptoms include muscle weakness, paralytic ileus, ECG abnormalities, decreased reflex response and, in severe form, respiratory paralysis, alkalosis and arrhythmia.

Diet and Cider Vinegar to Help Correct Potassium Deficiency

A high potassium diet has been shown to protect against heart disease, cancer and strokes. The human body contains more than twice the amount of potassium to sodium; however, the typical diet contains nearly twice as much sodium. Foods rich in potassium will provide the body cells with moisture-attracting potassium needed to win the contest with bacteria. Fruit, berries, edible leaves, edible roots, honey and apple cider vinegar are excellent sources of potassium.

One reason for the versatility of apple cider vinegar as a remedy is that it associates minerals with potassium. Apple cider vinegar carries over from the original apple the following minerals: phosphorus, chlorine, sodium, magnesium, calcium, sulfur, iron, fluorine, silicon and many trace minerals.

For medicinal purposes and for potassium supplement, the cider vinegar should be made from whole, mature apples. Some vinegars are made from apple peelings and cores. The label should tell you whether the cider vinegar was made from whole apples.

Besides eating fruits and vegetables high in potassium (bananas, dried apricots, peaches, cantaloupe, avocados, lima beans, potatoes, raw tomatoes, spinach, raw carrots, and asparagus), you can increase your intake of potassium by the use of paprika, honey/vinegar drinks, grape juice, apple juice and cranberry juice. The mineral content of grape juice is about 11.49 percent potassium. Grape juice quenches thirst promptly and the sugar is taken immediately into the circulation without undergoing any digestion process.

As you grow older, your intake of potassium should increase. Athletes or people who regularly exercise also need more potassium. A daily intake of at least four grams of potassium is recommended for these individuals, as up to three grams can be lost in one day by sweating (Senior Counselor 1991).

Potassium:Sodium

Both potassium and sodium have the ability to attract fluid. Within the body cells, potassium is responsible for drawing fluid into each cell. Outside the body cells sodium is responsible for the amount of fluid present. About 95 percent of the body's potassium is found within cells. Most of the sodium in the body is found outside the cells in the blood and interstitial fluid. Potassium and sodium carry on a lifelong battle over the supply of fluid.

Cells actually pump sodium out and potassium in. This pump is found in the membranes of all cells in the body. One of the functions of this pumping system is to prevent swelling. If sodium is not pumped out, water accumulates in the cell which may cause it to swell and ultimately burst.

The sodium-potassium pump also works to maintain the electrical charge within cells. This is particularly important to muscle and nerve cells. During nerve transmission and muscle contraction, potassium exits the cell and sodium enters, resulting in a change in electrical charge. This change is what causes a nerve impulse or muscle contraction. A potassium deficiency affects muscles and nerves first (Senior Counselor 1991).

Balance of Sodium to Potassium

The balance of sodium to potassium has a great impact on your health. Too much sodium in the diet can disrupt this balance. Numerous studies have shown that a low-potassium-high-sodium diet plays a major role in the development of cancer and cardiovascular disease (heart disease, high blood pressure, strokes, etc.).

Most Americans have a potassium-to-sodium ratio of less than 0.5. This means they ingest twice as much sodium as potassium. Researchers recommend a dietary potassium-to-sodium ratio of greater than 5 to maintain health. This is ten times higher than the average intake.

Apple cider vinegar is a potent source of potassium. Most fresh fruits and vegetables have a potassium-to-sodium ratio of at least 50:1. A natural diet rich in these foods can produce a potassium-to-sodium ratio greater than 100:1.

The Relationship of Potassium to Iron and Calcium

Lymph nodes can become enlarged when the lymph channels are blocked. Such a blockage can be caused by a precipitation of iron due to lack of potassium. If the blockage is the result of iron precipitation, you can correct the problem with an increased intake of potassium, and the glands should decrease in size.

The potassium and acetic acid in apple cider vinegar can affect calcium deposits in joints. Calcium enters into solution when it is in an acid liquid environment. Calcium leaves a solution when it is in an alkaline environment. What does this mean?

Blood is weakly alkaline or base. With an increase of alkalinity above normal, calcium is precipitated out of solution and deposited in the tissues. When you flood your blood with a natural acid, the potassium it contains dissolves into solution any calcium deposits. Drinking apple cider vinegar, cranberry juice or grape juice with meals will keep blood-vessel walls free from calcium deposits. Potassium controls the use of calcium in the body.

You can experiment for yourself. If there is calcium oxide in your water, indicated by calcium deposits on the sides of your pots, boil a solution of one cup of cider vinegar to a quart of water. The calcium deposits will dissolve into the solution. After water has been boiled, it will show an alkaline reaction. Calcium leaves a solution in an alkaline environment. Apple cider vinegar will dissolve an egg shell. Calcium enters into solution in an acid medium and is precipitated and deposited in an alkaline medium.

When foods are cooked in water, a reduction of potassium averages 70 percent in the case of carrots, onions, potatoes, squash and spinach; 60 percent for cauliflower, cabbage, peas, asparagus, string beans, brussel sprouts; 50 percent in corn, beets and tomatoes (Senior Counselor 1991).

From the Mayo Clinic article *Directions for the Planning Preparation of Diets Low in Content of Potassium* by Sister Mary Victory, B.S., Fellow in Nutrition, the Mayo Foundation, we learn that certain amounts of calcium and potassium are lost when the medium shifts its reaction from acid to alkaline.

Can You Over Dose on Potassium?

The estimated safe and adequate daily dietary intake of potassium as set by the Committee on Recommended Daily Allowances, is 1.9 to 5.6 grams. Eating fresh fruits and vegetables and adding cider vinegar to your diet are the best ways to meet the body's potassium needs. Supplementation is often necessary, especially for the elderly. Potassium salts are commonly prescribed by physicians in the dosage range of 1.5 to 3.0 grams per day. These salts do occasionally have side affects—nausea, vomiting, diarrhea and ulcers.

Some people cannot effectively excrete potassium, such as people with a kidney disease. They are likely to experience heart disturbances and other consequences of potassium toxicity. Generally, most people cannot take too much potassium (Senior Counselor 1991).

ADVERSE EFFECTS OF VINEGARS

In my research I have not found anything that indicates any type of adverse effect from the use of cider vinegar. I suggest that anything taken to excess can have an adverse effect, including drinking too much water. Reason and common sense must prevail.

Cider vinegar will shorten the life of your perm if you use it as a hair rinse. Drinking a lot of cider vinegar and water may cause you to urinate more frequently. If you consider frequent urination to be an aid in cleansing the body of toxins, then, it really would not be considered an adverse effect.

Vinegars made from wine or malt may contain small amounts of tyramine, a natural chemical produced when bacteria digest the proteins in grapes or grains in the making of beer or wine. Tyramine is a pressor amine, a chemical that constricts blood vessels and raises blood pressure. Under ordinary circumstances tyramine is broken down by enzymes in the body and then harmlessly excreted. However, if you are taking drugs to arrest depression of hypertension, monoamine oxidase (MAO) inhibitors, there may be a possible interaction between the wine or malt-based vinegars and the MAO inhibitors. This reaction may prevent elimination of the tyramine from the body with the result of an increase in blood pressure (Rinzler 1990). Remember, not all vinegars are the same.

CHAPTER 4

MEDICINAL USES OF CIDER VINEGAR

I am not a medical doctor and do not recommend cider vinegar as a medical panacea. Most of the remedies presented here come from books about folk medicine and from studies performed by doctors, such as Dr. Jarvis. The scientific evidence, in medical publications, is increasing about cider vinegar as a medicinal aid. There is no evidence that cider vinegar can do you any harm.

A natural high can be achieved through good health. Most people know that adequate exercise, sleep and a well-managed diet contribute to this process of good health. We also know that a positive attitude toward life and a spiritual path enhance this natural high. All these factors together prevent premature aging.

The first yardstick of your health is your urine. I discussed this to some degree in the Medical Research Chapter under Acid-Alkaline Balance. Sickness appears on an alkaline-urine background. It is not difficult, nor does it cost very much, to test your urine yourself. You should be able to obtain testing paper at your local health food store or at your pharmacy. Feelgoodfood.com makes pHydrion Vivid 5.5 to 8.0 testing paper which costs about $13.95 per dispenser. If your urine tests alkaline, cider vinegar can help to restore it to an acid reaction.

Apple cider vinegar contains minute quantities of minerals which help to adjust our metabolism or bodily processes. It helps make the body function normally. Whether too acid to too alkaline, your urine can be brought back to normal if you drink two teaspoons of cider vinegar in a glass of water with each meal. It is helpful to know why cider vinegar works, and the Medical Research Chapter will answer some of your questions.

In the following section on the medicinal uses of cider vinegar, the dosage is not stressed because it tends to be an individual matter. The dosages vary from one teaspoon of cider vinegar in an eight ounce glass of water to four ounces of cider vinegar in an eight ounce glass. Each person can experiment with what the correct amount might be for them. You could use the urine test to determine the proper dosage. Also, there is no guarantee that apple cider vinegar will work for everyone. If for any reason your body has an adverse reaction to cider vinegar, try taking small amounts of apple juice and in that way you will at least receive the healthful properties of the apple.

If you are going to use cider vinegar for medicinal purposes, you will want to be certain of the quality of the vinegar you are using. I have included a chapter on the organic brands currently on the market. If you do not feel confident about any of the brands, you have the option of making your own and, therefore, having complete control over the quality of your cider vinegar. There is a chapter in this book to help you get started in the production of your own cider vinegar. Read the chapter on Commercial Production and make your own decision.

The following is a list of common problems which have been cured or helped through the use of cider vinegar. Included in the list are aids or preparations. This very extensive list dynamically demonstrates the tremendous versatility of apple cider vinegar. I do not personally make any recommendations. The best advice is to talk with your physician and get his/her thoughts before trying any of the following folk remedies. There may not be a separate detailed description for each problem listed. If you have a problem included in the list but can find no further information on it, start with one teaspoon of cider vinegar in a glass of water with each meal.

Angina	Hepatitis
Antibiotic	Herbal bath
Antidote for alkaline poison	Hiccough
Arthritis/Aching joints	High blood pressure
Asthma	Hives
Auto-intoxication	Indigestion
Bad breath	Influenza
Birth control	Insect bites
Bladder infection	Insomnia

Blood clotting

Bronchitis

Burns

Bursitis

Chapped hands

Cold

Cold sores

Colic

Colitis

Colon problems

Constipation

Corns/Callouses

Coughs

Cramps

Dandruff

Diarrhea

Dizziness

Douche

Dysentery

Ear ache

Eczema

Expectorant

Eye problems

Facial neuralgia

Fainting

Fatigue

Itchy skin

Joint problems

Kidney problems

Laryngitis

Leg Pain

Lice

Liniments

Liver problems

Menstrual problems

Morning sickness

Mouth infections

Mucus problems

Nausea

Nerve problems

Neuralgia

Nose problems

Obesity

Osteoarthritis

Pancreatic problems

Paranasal sinusitis

Pimples

Pleurisy

Pneumonia

Poison ivy

Purification of body

Rash

Fever

Fingernail problems

Flu

Freckle removal

Gallbladder problems

Gallstones

Gout

Hair care

Hand care

Hay fever

Headaches

Heart

Heartburn

Hemorrhoids

Respiratory problems

Rheumatism

Ring worm

Round worm

Shingles

Sinusitis

Skin problems

Sore throat

Sprains

Strains

Teeth problems

Throat problems

Ulcers

Vaginal problems

Angina

Angina is a condition in which the arteries of the heart do not always pass enough blood. This may cause pain in the upper chest which often affects the left arm and neck. Your physician might give you nitroglycerin tablets which would give you almost immediate relief. Apple cider vinegar in water taken regularly will lessen the severity of the attack.

Antibiotic

Research has proven that a 5 percent concentration of acetic acid is lethal to many microorganisms. Lower concentrations have been found to be quite effective. A 1 percent solution is used prophylactically in surgical dressings, and a .25 percent solution is used in catheterization and irrigation of the bladder. Vaginal infections caused by Candida and Trichomonas are treated with douche solutions of .25 percent to 1 percent.

Cider vinegar was used to treat wounds in World War I and has been used as an antibiotic since Biblical times (Diggs 1989).

Arthritis/Aching joints

Hard calcium deposits fill up and cement joints, sometimes enlarging and crippling the joints. In the chapter on Medical Research relating to cider vinegar, it was explained how calcium precipitates out of a solution in an alkaline medium and back into solution in an acid medium. Apple cider vinegar helps to provide the acid medium to reduce calcium deposits in joints.

Dr. D.C. Jarvis recommends that two teaspoons of cider vinegar and two teaspoons of honey be mixed in a glass of water and taken with each meal or between meals. On Monday, Wednesday and Friday add one drop of iodine to the mixture at one meal. Take one kelp tablet at breakfast or at all three meals. Avoid wheat foods, cereals, white sugar, citrus fruits and muscle meats as these foods will produce an adverse reaction. He recommends this remedy for arthritis, osteoarthritis, bursitis and gout.

Look for control of symptoms, easing of pain and reduction in the development of the condition. Keep as mobile as possible and do not give up hope. If possible, add gentle massage therapy to your health maintenance program.

You can also experience some relief from the pain of arthritis by soaking for at least fifteen minutes a day in a bath of warm water to which 1-2 cups of cider vinegar have been added. As you soak, gently massage the sensitive areas yourself. Besides helping to alleviate the pain, the cider vinegar will provide your skin with the acid mantle it needs to be healthy (Jarvis 1958).

Asthma

Take two teaspoons of cider vinegar with two teaspoons of honey in water three times a day. Warm and sip this mixture before bed. Breathe deeply (Hanssen 1978).

Auto-intoxication

If you feel lethargic, it may be time to flush out some toxins which have accumulated in your system for one reason or another. Apple cider vinegar is an excellent preventative of auto-intoxication. Cider vinegar prevents this disease promoting condition because of its action on the liver. It has the power of detoxicating the poisons that accumulate in the organ and at the same time implementing their elimination from the body. Cider vinegar may be called a hepatic remedy. For proper elimination, pectin is necessary for binding. Pectin is an ingredient in cider vinegar to promote healthy action of the bowels. One of the best ways to introduce bulk foods into your system is to use bran in your diet for the needed bulk and roughage. Elimination organs can use your help. Cider vinegar is a good aid.

Bad breath

With the improvement of digestion through the use of cider vinegar, foods ingested will be more completely digested. There will be less food putrefaction and the resulting bad breath. Cider vinegar destroys the unwanted putrefaction bacteria in the digestive tract. Decomposition is the prime cause of many diseases. Cider vinegar is an agent which prevents decomposition.

Birth control
A solution of .25 percent to 1 percent cider vinegar has been used as a spermatocide (Diggs 1989).

Bladder infections
Eat a dish of raw tomatoes with cider vinegar and olive oil. Sip a glass of apple juice with one teaspoon of cider vinegar. Use this combination at least three times a week (Bragg 1989).

Blood clotting
Cider vinegar helps with the clotting of blood. It improves metabolism and helps with the assimilation of phosphate of potash, phosphate of iron and to some extent chloride of sodium in the blood (Scott 1982).

Bronchitis
Bronchitis can be treated naturally by using good judgment and perseverance in habits and diet. Smoking, crowds and alcohol should be avoided. Drink warm drinks. Herbal teas are highly recommended. The addition of apple cider vinegar, ginger or mineral water to hot baths is effective in breaking up bronchial congestion. Get plenty of fresh air and breathe deeply. Avoid citrus fruits because they make the body alkaline and tend to prolong the cleansing process. Cranberries, raw and

blended with honey and cider vinegar, are very helpful in cleansing the kidneys in this illness. Drink lots of honey and cider vinegar warm drinks to sooth the throat and bronchus (Malstrom 1977).

Burns

Use pure, undiluted cider vinegar to relieve the pain and soreness from minor sun burns. The relief is immediate. It takes the sting right out and will minimize any peeling. Cider vinegar also has an antiseptic quality. Concentrations of 5 percent have been found to be effective in treating extensive burns (Diggs 1989).

Bursitis—See Arthritis.

Chapped hands—See Skin problems.

Colds

Cider vinegar reduces the number of colds by building up the body in general. The cider vinegar-honey warm drink will help relieve many of the discomforts that accompany a cold. Take this drink particularly before going to bed. If you have a cough along with the cold, keep a honey-cider vinegar mixture near the bed for quick use during a coughing session. See coughs.

Colitis

Colitis is an inflammation of the mucous membrane of the colon. Take two teaspoons of cider vinegar and two teaspoons of honey in a glass of water three times a day.

Colon problems

You can minimize the chances of developing colitis, diverticulitis and perforated colon by the regular use of cider vinegar in your diet.

Constipation

The body is a self-healing and self-repairing organism. To help the body it is necessary to have regular bowel movements. Cider vinegar is not a cure but it is a great aid to heath in general. Make a tea of two tablespoons of flaxseed in two cups of boiling water and steep for fifteen minutes. Strain off the flaxseed and to the remaining liquid add one teaspoon of cider vinegar to a cup of this tea. Drink this on an empty stomach. Use this drink until you get a good daily bowel movement (Bragg 1989).

Another remedy suggested is to try a drink of cider vinegar and water upon rising and with each meal. Before retiring take a warm cup of honey, vinegar and water. Take two tablespoons of bran each day for one month. If you try this remedy and the condition does not improve, see your physician (Hanssen 1978).

Corns and callouses

Soak the corns or callouses in warm water for ten minutes and then dry. Apply undiluted cider vinegar to them and leave it on for ten minutes. Wash off and dry again.

Coughs

Drink a glass of water with four teaspoons of cider vinegar added to it. Sip the drink slowly when the cough is aggravated.

Cramps

When precipitated acid crystals get into the circulation of the legs and other parts of the body, they cause severe cramps. Drink two teaspoons of cider vinegar with two teaspoons of honey in a glass of water three times a day. The precipitated acid crystals will then enter into a solution form and pass out of the body by way of the kidneys and other organs of elimination.

Apply compresses of cider vinegar to the area of the cramp, spasm or tension. Use several cups of cider vinegar in your bath water. Drink a cup of cider vinegar-honey-water drink before retiring to reduce the frequency of attacks (Hanssen 1978; Buchman 1980; Bragg 1989).

Dandruff

You can use cider vinegar undiluted or in a water solution as a hair rinse. It will remove any alkaline residue left behind by your shampoo and will provide the scalp with the acid mantle the skin needs for health. It will leave your hair clean, softer and dandruff free. If you don't like the fragrance of cider vinegar as a hair rinse, you can add herbs to it to create the fragrance you do like. Check the section on cosmetic uses.

Diarrhea

When you have diarrhea, you lose lots of fluid. You will need to increase your intake of fluids at least two to three extra pints a day. To each half pint add one teaspoon of cider vinegar. This drink can be taken along with any other treatment prescribed (Hanssen 1978).

Dizziness

Check your urine for an alkaline reaction. To prevent dizziness use the apple cider vinegar mixture of two tablespoons to a glass of water. Do not expect to be free from dizziness the next day or forever because you took several drinks. You should, however, notice some lessening of the dizziness at the end of two weeks if you take the cider drink regularly with each meal. By the end of the month, you should notice a considerable improvement. When the urine reaction shifts back to acid, your dizziness will have diminished or will have disappeared altogether (Jarvis 1958).

Douche—See Vaginal problems.

Ear ache—Swimmer's Ear

The pH of a normal ear should be acidic. Warm the vinegar and put some in the sore ear. Allow the vinegar to stay in the ear about fifteen seconds and then turn your head so the excess can run out. Within fourteen hours the ear should have improved. The organisms that thrive in the dark, warm, wet ear canal cannot thrive in an acid environment.

Dr. Irving L. Ochs demonstrated that the acetic acid in cider vinegar acts as a bactericidal (kills bacteria). He treated external otitis, a severe form of ear infection with cider vinegar.

Eczema

Eczema arises from a deficiency of potassium chloride in the system. Take the cider vinegar drink with meals and use diluted cider vinegar applied directly to the skin. Cider vinegar baths will also help to alleviate this condition.

Expectorant

A honey-cider vinegar drink will promote expectoration and freedom of breathing (Diggs 1989).

Eye problems

Cider vinegar slows down or retards development of cataract. Cataracts occur when the body is lacking in cell salts, fluoride of calcium, phosphate of potash, silica and vitamin C.

Facial neuralgia

Test your urine. You will probably find that you get an alkaline reaction (the test paper turns blue). You need to shift the reaction to acid. Drink a glass of water with one teaspoon of cider vinegar each hour for three hours. Sip the acidified water throughout the day.

All acids do not produce the same effect in the body. Diluted hydrochloric acid taken four times a day for a period of two weeks will increase the pain of arthritis in the small joints of the hands and feet; whereas, one teaspoon of cider vinegar in a glass of water four times a day will result in relief from the pain in the same period of time (Hanssen 1978).

Fainting

One possible cause for fainting would be a potassium deficiency. You can work to correct this deficiency by increasing your intake of foods high in potassium as detailed in the

Medical Research chapter. Cider vinegar is a potent source of potassium (Bragg 1989).

<u>Fatigue–Chronic</u>

Chronic fatigue is a warning sign that you are out of step with the laws of nature. You can recognize chronic fatigue when a night's sleep does not remove the sense of tiredness, and you are tired when you start your day. Everything you do seems to take a lot of effort. You have no drive or initiative. You have spells of deep discouragement.

First, become aware of the amount of sound sleep you are getting at night. If you think that you might not be getting enough sleep, start with this area of the problem. Reserve energy is stored in the body by hours of body rest, sleep, freedom from worry and avoidance of foods that produce an alkaline urine reaction.

To help relax you before bed take a cider vinegar bath. Add about two cups or so to your bath water and relax in the water for at least fifteen minutes. Massage yourself in the water. Avoid using soap because soap is alkaline and helps to create in your body the very fatigue you wish to get rid of. You can tell if your skin is alkaline because it will normally be dry and itchy. Wash with a mixture of cider vinegar and water to maintain the normal acid skin reaction.

Before going to bed, drink a cup of warm honey-vinegar mixture. Honey acts as a sedative to the body and is one of the best remedies to produce sleep. Twenty minutes after you have taken this drink, it is in the blood stream.

Another honey-vinegar mixture sleep remedy suggests that you prepare a jar of three teaspoons of cider vinegar to a cup of honey. Keep the jar in the bedroom and take two teaspoons of this mixture when preparing to go to bed. You will be asleep within a half hour after getting into bed. In the case of extreme wakefulness, it may take several doses. This treatment is superior to sleeping pills, is a harmless treatment and can be taken indefinitely.

There are several foods you should avoid eating if you have chronic fatigue. Wheat is a primary problem. It produces weariness and weakness. Start to eat more things from the sea because one reason for fatigue is need for more iodine and other minerals. Baked beans with cider vinegar is excellent for someone troubled with chronic fatigue (Jarvis 1958).

Fingernail problems

Your fingernails can tell you much about your digestive system. White spots in the nails may be the result of ineffective use of the calcium in your diet. Deep ridges and indentations in the nails, along with a white coating on the tongue, indicate long term digestive problems. Apple cider vinegar can help both the nails and the digestive problems. Start by drinking the cider vinegar drink between meals. Give yourself at least one month before making any evaluations on the result of this treatment.

Freckle removal

Drink one teaspoon of cider vinegar in a glass of water upon rising and regularly apply undiluted 5 percent acid cedar vinegar to the freckles you want removed.

Gallbladder problems

If you have a gallbladder or liver problem, you should avoid choleretics, agents that stimulate the liver to increase production of bile, and cholagogues, agents that stimulate the gallbladder and bilary duct to discharge bile and increase your body's excretion of cholesterol. Avoid ginger, peppermint, oregano and turmeric (Rinzler 1990).

Gallstones

The recommended remedies to assist you in passing gallstones are pretty much in agreement with each other. No food is eaten during this process. You begin with a flush, drinking just apple juice for one week. After the one week, drink an eight ounce glass of 1/3 olive oil, 2/3 apple juice and 1 tablespoon of cider vinegar. You may drink apple juice throughout the day but no water. On the second day you take this same drink mixture twice during the day. On the third day eat a salad of raw cabbage, carrots, celery, beets, tomatoes and lettuce with cedar vinegar and olive oil. Eat a dish of steamed greens such as spinach, kale or other leafy greens. The apple juice will soften the stones to make them pass more easily. The olive oil causes the gallbladder to spasm and start the passage. They say you should find gallstones in your bowel movement.

Before you try this remedy, consult with your physician because gallstones are not all composed of the same things–some are cholesterol deposits and others have a higher mineral content. Passing gallstones can be a very painful process. If you try this, I suggest that you have a friend or relative with you to assist if there is a problem. Warm compresses and massage to the sensitive areas will help. This treatment will not dissolve the stones, only soften them (Malstrom 1977; Bragg 1989).

Gout—See Arthritis.

Hair care

Loss of hair is an indication of faulty metabolism. Taking the cider vinegar drink of one teaspoon of cider vinegar to a glass of water may stop hair loss and help hair growth. You might also add one teaspoon of horseradish to your two main meals of the day. Loss of hair is primarily due to deficiency of the tissue salts sodium chloride in minute doses, calcium phosphate and silicic oxide. Sulphate of lime may also be lacking. Cider vinegar can re-establish the balance needed for healthy hair (Scott 1982).

A solution of cider vinegar is an excellent hair rinse because it removes the alkaline residue left by your shampoo. You will have squeaky—clean hair and at the same time this rinse will restore the natural acid mantle necessary for healthy skin and hair. The rinse will also help if there is any dandruff problem.

If you have a perm, however, you might want to dilute the solution considerably because cider vinegar can shorten the life of your perm.

Hand care—See Skin problems.

Headache

A headache is a warning signal that something is wrong somewhere in the body. It can be an emotional headache as the result of stress and problems. It can be caused by trouble in the gallbladder, liver, kidneys or other important organs.

Check your urine for acid-alkaline reaction. If it is alkaline, you can aid the kidneys in getting the urine back to the normal acid reaction with cider vinegar. Besides drinking the cider vinegar drink of vinegar and water, put equal parts of cider and water in a pan and heat over the stove. Put a towel over your head and breathe in the fumes. Take at least fifty breaths. A chronic headache may be gone in thirty-five to forty minutes (Bragg 1989).

Treat yourself to a cider vinegar bath and self-massage. The warm water and cider vinegar will relax the muscles and relieve soreness. Work the back of your neck and shoulders while relaxing in the water. Try to stay in this vinegar bath at least fifteen minutes. Splash some of the bath water on your face. Soak a cloth in vinegar, wring it out, fold and apply to the forehead.

Healing agent

The healing process can be speeded up by taking one or two teaspoons of cider vinegar in a half or whole glass of water with each meal. Do this for two to three weeks prior to any surgical operation. It will minimize bleeding and speed the healing (Scott 1982).

Heart

The heart is a muscle. It uses large amounts of potassium and must have a continuous, constant supply of potassium for power and energy. Before any form of exercise, including taking a walk, drink a cider vinegar drink of one to two teaspoons of cider vinegar in a glass of water. Try to drink this mixture three times a day between meals (Bragg 1989).

Heartburn

This condition can be lessened by including a cider vinegar drink with each meal. Sip the drink throughout the meal. This remedy should work unless there is some serious disorder in the stomach.

Hemorrhoids

Hemorrhoids occur for various reasons–pregnancy, constipation, strain. They can be internal or external and are dilated veins in swollen anal tissue. They can be very painful and irritating.

Apple cider vinegar can be used to reduce the itching. Repeat the application every night or when you feel it is necessary. In three weeks the swelling and itching should be gone. In addition to external application, drink the cider vinegar drink of one teaspoon of cider vinegar to a glass of water at least three times a day.

Herbal bath—See Cosmetic uses.

Hiccoughs

Drink a glass of water with one teaspoon of cider vinegar in it with each meal (Scott 1982).

High blood pressure

High blood pressure and hypertension are a growing health problem. They are associated with three-fourths of annual deaths which are the result of heart and kidney disease. Some times high blood pressure is considered a disease and other times a symptom of a disease. From medical literature on the subject, the mechanism seems clear by which blood pressure is elevated to essential hypertension. In the early stages of hypertension the constriction of the arterioles is easily reversible and during sleep the blood pressure returns to normal, indicating a relaxation of the arterioles (small blood vessels). Per my research, high blood pressure appears to have two main explanations. One attributes the condition to over activity of the sympathetic nervous system, which organizes the body for fight or flight and causes widespread constriction of the arterioles. The second explanation is that chemical substances circulate in the blood and produce a narrowing of the arterioles.

High blood pressure is not a fixed physiologic constant. It will vary with physical activity, rest, ingestion of food, weather, pain, nervous stress and strain. Weather is especially significant. Blood pressure is highest in cold weather, lowest in warm weather. The blood is always alkaline in reaction. If the alkalinity is increased, the blood thickens and precipitates its solids in tiny flakes. The walls of the tiny blood vessels in the arterial tree allow the fluid part of the blood to pass. But thickened blood will not pass through as easily. The little flakes plug some of the tiny blood vessels with a result of a backing up of the blood, resulting in an increase in blood pressure.

To correct this, increase your daily intake of acid. You can do this by eating apples, grapes, cranberries or drinking their juices. Take two teaspoons of cider vinegar in a glass of water three times a day. Balance your intake of carbohydrates and protein. Exchange wheat food for corn. Eliminate common table salt. Honey is a magnet for water and eaten with each meal it will draw excess fluid from the blood, lowering blood pressure and alleviating any tension disturbing the nervous system (Jarvis 1958).

Hives

Make a paste of three parts flour or corn starch to one part cider vinegar. Apply this mixture to the affected area (Harris 1968).

Indigestion

If you suffer from indigestion, heartburn, gas or bloating, you may not have enough hydrochloric acid in your stomach. If you find that by drinking the cider vinegar drink your indigestion is relieved, you can be almost certain that this is the case.

Digestion and absorption of nutriments continues in the small intestine where enzymes and essential bacteria help to break down food into substances which can be absorbed by the body. These bacteria appear to find much benefit from cider vinegar which contains both potassium and acetic acid in apparently balanced amounts. The high potassium content may be the factor in the settling effect obtained by drinking the cider vinegar drink–one to two teaspoons of cider vinegar to a glass of water (Hanssen 1978).

Before each meal, take one tablespoon of water to which you have added two drops of cider vinegar. Hold it in your mouth for a few seconds to start the salivary glands working. Weak saliva can also cause gas, heartburn and bloating as the starch in your diet need this saliva to begin digestion. Cider vinegar before a meal will help the digestive fluids flow faster (Bragg 1989).

It is important to a healthy digestive system to have fiber daily. The simplest way to get this fiber is to consume two tablespoons of bran each day which can be mixed with a little of the cider vinegar drink or added to your food. The results are remarkable if continued on a regular basis (Hanssen 1978).

If you believe that your indigestion problem is the result of insufficient digestive acids, cider vinegar and honey (one tablespoon of each) plus a cup of water may also be used several times a day to help re-balance the body (Buchman 1980).

Insect bites

Apply undiluted cider vinegar directly to the bite. It will take away the sting and help it heal sooner.

Insomnia

Before going to bed, take a cider vinegar bath to relax. Stay in the bath for at least fifteen minutes. Prepare a jar of three teaspoons of cider vinegar to a cup of honey. Keep this jar in the bedroom and take two teaspoons of the mixture when preparing to go to bed. You will be asleep within a half hour after getting into bed. In the case of extreme wakefulness, it may take several does and some counting of blessings. This treatment is superior to sleeping pills because it can be taken indefinitely and is a harmless treatment (Jarvis 1958).

Itchy skin

Soak in a cider vinegar bath and drink the cider vinegar drink three times a day. See skin problems.

Joint problems

When the body begins to creak and crack, this could be a sign of a deficiency. Too much table salt disturbs the metabolism of the body. Cut down on the consumption of table salt or eliminate it completely.

The remedy for this condition is to drink a cider vinegar-water drink with each meal. You should notice a positive change in about one month. If the deposits in the joints are calcium, it will take longer. Stay active and take cider vinegar baths (Scott 1982).

Kidney problems

Taking a drink of two teaspoons of cider vinegar in a glass of water with each meal will help the kidney problems. If there is an inflammation in the kidneys called pyelitis, noted by pus cells in the urine, this drink will clear up the condition. Some kidney stones can be dissolved by using cider vinegar. Use cider vinegar on your raw vegetable salads. Eat prunes, raisins and apples (Jarvis 1958).

Laryngitis

Drink a half a glass of water with one teaspoon of cider vinegar every hour for several hours. A little honey may be added to this mixture.

Leg pains

Soak in a warm cider vinegar bath for at least fifteen minutes and self-massage the sensitive areas.

Lice

Use cider vinegar directly and undiluted from the bottle. Rub it into the scalp and make sure it reaches the base of the hair strands. Leave it on the head for fifteen minutes and then rinse out. Shampoo and rinse again with cider vinegar. This should kill the lice. If it does not kill all of them, repeat this treatment several times until they are gone.

Liniments

Add one tablespoon of cayenne pepper to a pint of warm cider vinegar and let sit for one hour. Stir, strain and label the bottle. Before applying this liniment, warm the affected bruised area with warm, wet packs. Gently rub in a small amount of the liniment twice an hour for two to three hours and apply a hot water bottle or cover with heavy flannel (Harris 1968).

Another liniment recipe is a mixture of cider vinegar and turpentine. Mix one egg together with seven ounces of turpentine and two teaspoons of oil of lemon until thoroughly mixed. Add cider vinegar (2 and 2/3 ounces) and water until you have sixteen ounces. Shake vigorously. Shake this remedy well before using it (Harris 1968).

Liver problems—See Gallbladder problems.

Menstrual problems

If menstruation is profuse, the cider vinegar drink will reduce the flow of blood by about 50 percent. The amount of clots will also decrease. If, however, taking the drink delays the onset for a few days, discontinue taking the drink for three or four days prior to the expected menstrual date (Scott 1982).

If you have severe cramps during your menstruation, soak in a bath of water and cider vinegar. This will warm the blood which can then flow more easily.

Morning sickness—See Nausea.

Mouth infections

Mouth ulcers and sores will benefit from a mouth wash made of one teaspoon of cider vinegar in water after you brush your teeth in the morning and at night.

Mucus problems

Discontinue eating dairy products, eggs and meat. Drink plenty of cider vinegar drink (one to two teaspoons to a glass of water). Make a drink of cider vinegar and honey to your taste and drink throughout the day. Paprika is a rich source of potassium. Along with cider vinegar, drink apple juice and grape juice. Sip the drinks slowly (Bragg 1989).

If you have wetness of the eyes, seepage from sinuses or watery discharge from the nose, one teaspoon of cider vinegar in a glass of water will clear up these conditions in one to two weeks. Avoid citrus fruits and wheat products. Replace wheat with rye or corn products (Jarvis 1958).

Nausea

Take one teaspoon of cider vinegar in a glass of water. If this helps the condition, continue the treatment. If not, discontinue. You should try it at least for a day, sipping the drink throughout the day.

Nerve problems

Twitching of the eyelids or corners of the mouth is called a tic. If you have nervous tics, take one teaspoon of cider vinegar in a glass of equal parts grape juice and water. Take this drink in the middle of the morning and mid-afternoon (Scott 1982).

For general well-being and to relax, a warm cider vinegar bath is highly recommended. This will benefit your skin as well as your nerves. Take time for yourself away from stressful situations–walk, swim, stretch, meditate. Take care of yourself and your health. You don't really appreciate your health until it's gone. Start take care now before it's gone.

Nose problems

Cider vinegar will reduce the number of colds you will have by building up your body in general. Take vitamin C also. For a stuffy nose, use cider vinegar as an inhalant by warming a diluted solution of it over the stove. Cover your head with a towel and inhale the warm rising steam (Scott 1982).

Because cider vinegar is an astringent, it is worth trying in the case of persistent nose bleeding (Hanssen 1978).

For watery discharge from the nose, take one teaspoon of cider vinegar in a glass of water. This condition should clear up in one to two weeks. Avoid citrus fruits and wheat products (Jarvis 1958).

Pancreatic problems

Malfunctioning of organs such as the liver and gallbladder, which are closely allied with the pancreas, may precipitate pancreatic problems. Duodenal ulcers, systemic infections, hydrochloric acid deficiency, lack of chromium in the diet—all may adversely affect the pancreas. A person with pancreatitis (inflammation of the pancreas) suffers from symptoms of acid indigestion, discomfort, nausea, pain and gas. Stools may be bulky and pale, reflecting poor digestion, especially of fats. When the pancreas is not secreting the proper amounts of enzymes, digestion problems occur. One can become weak and lose weight with severe malabsorption of their food. Diarrhea may also accompany this problem. Some things which can contribute to this problem are sugar, white flour, preservatives, milk products, meats, overly-processed foods and wrong food combinations (Malstrom 1977).

A diet high in raw vegetables and pancreatic enzymes are mandatory for a person with a weak pancreas. Apple cider vinegar and honey are a must. Because zinc prolongs the effect of insulin on blood sugar, foods rich in zinc and chromium should be included in the diet—pumpkin seeds, nuts, grains, seeds, green vegetables and molasses. Other beneficial herbs are uva ursi, cayenne, golden seal, juniper berries and Jerusalem artichokes (Malstrom 1977).

Paranasal sinusitis

Check your urine. It may be alkaline. You can shift the reaction to acid and relieve the pain by taking one teaspoon of cider vinegar to a glass of water every hour for seven hours (Hanssen 1978).

Pimples—See Skin problems.

Plague

The legend of the four thieves is fascinating history. The discovery of the following recipe is attributed to four thieves during a devastating bubonic plague. The thieves had been taking things from plague-ridden homes. They were caught and brought before a French judge in Marseilles. The judge asked how they had managed to steal things from infested homes and not be affected by the plague.

"We drank a vinegar drink every few hours," they answered. In return for giving up their recipe, they were given their freedom (Buchman 1980).

Vinegar of the Four Thieves
    2 quarts apple cider vinegar
    2 T lavender
    2 T rosemary
    2 T sage
    2 T wormwood
    2 T rue
    2 T mint
    2 T garlic buds

Combine the dried herbs and steep them in cider vinegar for two weeks in the sun. Strain, bottle and label. Add several cloves of garlic and then close the lid. When the garlic has steeped for several days, strain them out. Melt wax around the lid to preserve the contents or add four ounces of glycerine for preservation (Rose 1972).

This mixture can be used in diluted solutions as a body wash or added to your bath. It is an aromatic, antibacterial wash for floors, walls, sinks, bedsteads, pots, pans, sickrooms, bathrooms and kitchens.

Internally, the dose is a teaspoon at a time in water, no more than one tablespoon per hour. This drink acts as a preventative during flu epidemics.

Modern Anti-epidemic Cider Vinegar
1 quart apple cider vinegar
1 pound garlic buds for 8 ounces of juice
8 oz. Comfrey root
4 oz. Oak bark
4 oz. Marshmallow root
4 oz. Mullein flowers
4 oz. Rosemary flowers
4 oz. Lavender flowers
4 oz. Wormwood
4 oz. Black walnut leaves
12 oz. Glycerine

First soak each herb in clean spring water for a day. Simmer each herb separately for ten minutes. Steep for a half hour. Strain out material and simmer and reduce until each herb is concentrated. Press garlic buds into an eight-ounce concentrated juice. Add twelve ounces of glycerine to preserve it. Mix all ingredients together, bottle and label.

During any epidemic take one to three teaspoons a day. If a family member is ill with a communicable disease, take one teaspoon every hour. Dilute the solution with water if you find it too strong to take or add the teaspoon to a hot herbal tea (Rose 1972).

Pleurisy
A vinegar-honey drink will treat pleuritic affections (Diggs 1989).

Pneumonia

The treatment recommended for bronchitis will also work for pneumonia.

Poison Ivy

Apply cider vinegar undiluted to the affected area and soak in a cool bath of cider vinegar and water. Use about two cups to a bath tub of water.

Purification of the body

Toxic poisons are the cause of many troubles in the body. Certain toxic wastes that are harmful to the body are rendered harmless by acetolysis, a substance in cider vinegar. You can rid the body of toxic wastes by cell purification. Every ninety days a new blood stream is built in the body by the food you eat, the liquid you drink and the air you breathe. From the blood stream the body cells are made and nourished. Besides drinking a cider vinegar-water drink three times a day, include tomato juice once or twice daily (Bragg 1989).

Rashes

Try an undiluted solution of cider vinegar applied directly to the rash. Soak in an apple cider vinegar bath. If the condition does not improve in several days, discontinue treatment and consult your physician.

Respiratory problems

If the respiratory problem is an inflammation of the mucous membrane, put a couple of inches of cider vinegar in a small stainless steel or enamel saucepan and simmer gently. Inhale the vapors for five to ten minutes. This will bring relief for up to eight hours.

Rheumatism

A rub for rheumatism made of one teaspoon of oil of wintergreen and one pint of apple cider vinegar is useful on inflamed rheumatic joints, stiff swollen joints, swellings and sprains. Soak a cloth in this preparation and wring out. Apply the cloth to the affected area. The wintergreen will bring blood to the surface of the skin. The apple cider vinegar eases the pain and helps to release some of the toxins. Check the skin for sensitivity to the wintergreen (Rose 1972).

Shingles

Shingles are usually experienced as burning pain, usually along the path of a nerve. Dab undiluted cider vinegar regularly on the sore areas. This should give you relief. Repeat as the pain returns (Hanssen 1978).

Shingles are related to a nervous condition. You might want to add to your health routine an evening bath of cider vinegar. Relax and soak for at least fifteen minutes and do a little self-massage in the areas where you feel tight.

Sinusitis

This problem may appear as too much mucus in the sinuses. Sugar, white flour, meat, eggs and salt are mucus producing, along with dairy products. You can help improve your condition by eating raw vegetables supplemented with vitamins

A, C and D. It is important to cleanse the colon to clear up the sinuses. Drink the cider vinegar drink of one teaspoon of vinegar to a glass of water with each meal (Malstrom 1977).

Skin problems

Steam your face over a pan of boiling or simmering water with a towel over your head. This will open the pores. As an alternative you can just lay back and relax with a hot towel on your face. After the pores have opened, pat cider vinegar in diluted solution on the skin with a cotton ball to remove the loosened dirt. Repeat twice and then pat the cider vinegar on to close the pores and tone the skin. This steam cleaning should be done once a week. The treatment is good for skin blemishes and pimples. Cider vinegar will restore the natural acid mantle necessary for healthy skin. Soaps leave an alkaline residue which is not the natural nature of your skin. Keep the vinegar away from your eyes (Bragg 1989).

Sore throat—See Throat problems.

Sprains

Cider vinegar compresses often relieve a sprain. The following is a particular liniment recipe for sprains, strains, swollen joints and arthritic pain. Before applying this liniment, check the skin for sensitivity. Mix together one teaspoon cayenne pepper, six drops oil of pine, and one pint of apple cider vinegar. This mixture can be used at body temperature or heated. Apply directly to the sprain and wrap it (Rose 1972).

Strains—See Sprains.

Sunburn

Cider vinegar is an excellent treatment for sunburn. It is not a preventative. Apply the cider vinegar directly from the bottle to the sunburn. It will immediately relieve the burn, sting and prevent peeling. Soak for a minimum of fifteen minutes in a cool bath to which two cups of cider vinegar have been added. If the sunburn is severe with blisters already formed, consult your physician.

Teeth problems

Teeth should be brushed with a solution of one teaspoon cider vinegar in a glass of water at night and in the morning. After brushing, use this mixture as a mouth wash. Mouth ulcers and sores benefit from this mouth wash (Hanssen 1978).

Throat problems

The following treatment has been used to cure a streptococci sore throat in twenty-four hours. Make a mix of one teaspoon of cider vinegar to a glass of water. Gargle this solution every hour and then swallow the solution. Swallow a second mouthful. Swallowing allows the solution to reach all parts of the lower throat. As the soreness lessens, increase the time between gargling (Jarvis 1958).

Make an apple cider vinegar compress and apply it to the throat area. Bind the compress with a piece of wool or a wool sock. This will also help relieve he most painful of sore throats (Buchman 1980).

Ulcers

Some of the most frequent stomach and small intestine complaints turn out to be ulcers, which are caused by poor diet and stress. The resultant pain and distress can cause both oral and rectal bleeding. One half teaspoon of capsicum (cayenne pepper) mixed with cider vinegar and water taken two or three times a day can give amazing relief and aid healing.

An ulcer diet is recommended for healing any and all parts of the digestive system. For the first two or three weeks, eat raw vegetables blended into a pulp along with green drinks. After that, add fruit juices and whole soft vegetables and fruits until you can eat all whole vegetables. Stay on this diet for three to four months. In making your green drinks, consider adding spiralina which is a complete protein.

Stay away from refined sugars, white flour products, mucus-forming foods such as dairy products, highly processed foods, all alcoholic beverages, soft drinks and other irritating foods.

You will also want to increase the friendly bacteria in the small intestine. Use acidophilus or buttermilk to help build up these needed beneficial bacteria (Malstrom 1977).

Vaginal problems

Cider vinegar has been used for many generations as a feminine vaginal douche. Vaginal infections caused by candida and trichomonas are treated with douche solutions of .25 percent to 1 percent. These solutions are also used as a spermatocide (Diggs 1989).

For general douching purposes you might prefer a scented douche. If so, mix together ½ ounce of the following: lavender, rosemary, mint, thyme. To these dried herbs add one quart of cider vinegar. Steep this mixture for two weeks, shaking daily. Strain and filter the liquid through filter paper and bottle for use. When you want to use it, add ½ to one cup of the scented vinegar to a douche bag and fill with warm water (Rose 1972).

Warts

Apply cider vinegar full strength to the warts. Leave on the application. You may want to put the cider vinegar in a cotton swab and use tape to keep the swab in place. Rub the warts also with fresh cut apples.

Wasp sting

Apply cider vinegar directly to the sting. Reapply if it continues to sting. Secure a small compress of cider vinegar to the sting until you feel relief.

Weight problems

Apple cider vinegar will help you to achieve a normal weight. It improves the functioning and adjustment of the body so that there is efficient use made of the food you eat. Dr. Jarvis, Paul Bragg and others claim this to be true. You become satisfied and content with the correct amount of food for you. The cider vinegar can do much for you, but you must provide yourself with a proper, nutritious diet. If you feel you present diet is okay, no change in your daily food intake will be necessary except to avoid foods that you know will increase fat deposits in the body.

If you want to improve your diet, eliminate over-refined foods, sugar, salt and wheat products. Eat green vegetables and fresh fruit daily. You must include protein in your diet because it builds muscles and repairs cells. You can get your protein from nuts, soy beans, milk, eggs, cheese, fish and lean meat.

The loss of weight will be gradual. Start your day with two teaspoons of cider vinegar in a glass of water. The cider vinegar will make it possible to burn the fat in the body instead of store it. Sip a mixture of two teaspoons of cider vinegar with water with each meal and chew your food thoroughly. This modifies the desire to over eat and also promotes digestion. The average weight loss per week should be one and a half pounds. This will continue until you reach your proper weight (Scott 1982).

If you are under weight, the cider vinegar drink will also help you to arrive at your normal weight.

CHAPTER 5

OTHER USES OF CIDER VINEGAR

COOKING AND PRESERVING

Although man learned to make cheese and wine some two thousand years before the birth of Christ and maintain a yeast culture to raise his daily bread, the phenomena of fermentation remained a mystery for many years.

Though not understood, fermentation was responsible for the preservation of foods in vinegar. Though the pleasing acidity of limes, lemons and wood berries was familiar not only to the cave man and the tree dweller but to citizens of the ancient world, it was not until the alcohol in neglected wine changed to acetic acid that vinegar was discovered. The very name is derived from vin aigre, or sour wine, and like salt, vinegar proved to be a most successful preservative. In Egypt and Greece flowers, herbs, roots and vegetables were preserved in vinegar. Figs, apples, plums, cherries and pears were selected with great care and preserved in a mixture of vinegar and honey.

Meat and fish were preserved in salt and vinegar. Apicius taught the ancients to cover pieces of pork with a paste of salt, vinegar and honey. Pickled foods were agreeable additions to daily meals and helped to satisfy the increasing craving in civilized nations for a more varied diet.

COOKING AND PRESERVING

I am sure there are many recipes using cider vinegar. This book, however, is not primarily a cookbook. I have included some recipes just for your interest.

General uses

Baked beans: Soak beans overnight in cider vinegar and water instead of just water.

Rice: For an interesting flavor, try soaking 3/4 cup of rice in some cider vinegar before cooking.

Pies: When you make apple pie, use cider vinegar instead of water to moisten the crust mixture. You might also try adding a few drops on top of the apples before covering the crust.

Baked apples: Try adding cider vinegar to them while they are baking.

Soups: Add cider vinegar to your pea and onion soups.

Applesauce: Cider vinegar and honey add an interesting taste to applesauce.

Gravy: Add cider vinegar to your beef gravy.

Fish: Bake fish in vinegar and water.

No amount of cider vinegar is given in the above suggestions. Try a teaspoon or so and use your own judgment how much is best for you and the particular dish (Orton 1973).

Too sweet or salty: To save a dish that tastes too sweet or too salty after you've mixed the ingredients, add a dash of cider vinegar (Heinz 1989).

Revive vegetables: Vegetables that look wilted can be revived by soaking them in cold water to which one tablespoon of vinegar as been added.

Stronger gelatin: To make your gelatin stand up when temperatures rise, add a teaspoon of vinegar to your gelatin recipe.

Hard-Boiled eggs: Add two tablespoons of cider vinegar per quart of water before boiling your eggs to prevent cracking. The shells will also peel off easier.

Firmer, whiter fish: Soak your filet or seafood steak for 20 minutes in one quart of water and two tablespoons of vinegar.

Easy Buttermilk: Add a tablespoon of vinegar to a cup of milk and let stand five minutes to thicken.

Fluffy white rice: Add a teaspoon of vinegar to the boiling water. Your rice will be less sticky.

Salad Dressing Recipes

Basic Cider Vinegar/Oil Dressing:
½ C olive oil
1/4 C apple cider vinegar
3 cloves minced garlic
½ tsp honey
Mix these ingredients together in a glass jar and store in the refrigerator. Season with additional herbs, salt and pepper as you desire.

Honey/Celery Seed Dressing:
1 C olive oil
1/3 C cider vinegar
1 tsp celery seeds
3 T honey
1/4 tsp paprika
1 tsp dry mustard

Simple Greek Dressing:
1 C olive oil
1/4 C cider vinegar
½ tsp salt
1–2 oz crumbled feta cheese

Cabbage or Fresh Fruit Dressing:
1 C mayonnaise
1/4 C cider vinegar
½ C plain yogurt
2 T honey

Tomato/Garlic Dressing:
1 C tomato juice
3 cloves garlic
4 T safflower oil
4 T cider vinegar
½ tsp basil
Honey to taste
Mix these ingredients in a blender.

Creamy Italian Dressing:
1/3 C water
1/4 C cider vinegar
1 T honey
1 egg
½ tsp celery seeds
1/8 tsp dry mustard
1 large clove garlic
1 tsp tarragon vinegar
1 tsp salt
½ tsp black pepper
1 C olive oil

Green Salad Dressing:
1 C olive oil
½ C cider vinegar
1 C chopped fresh parsley
1 small green onion, chopped
2 T Peeled and grated ginger root
1/3 C honey
1/8 tsp basil
1/4 tsp curry powder
1/4 tsp dry mustard
1/8 tsp salt
pinch of black pepper

Lemon/Parsley Salad Dressing:
1 C olive oil
4 tsp cider vinegar
½ C Lemon juice
2 C fresh parsley
½ tsp marjoram
1/3 C chopped green bell peppers
1 tsp salt
dash of black pepper.

Tamari Salad Dressing:
1 C safflower oil
½ C cider vinegar
1/4 C tamari
1/4 C honey

Poppy Seed Dressing:

½ C water

1/4 to ½ C honey to taste

1/4 C cider vinegar

2 T dry mustard

3 T chopped onions

1 T poppy seeds

1 tsp salt

1 ½ C safflower oil

Cardamom Cream Dressing:

4 egg yolks

1/4 C cider vinegar

1 T sugar

1 T butter

1/4 tsp dry mustard

1/8 tsp ground cardamom

1/4 tsp salt

½ pint heavy cream

1 C miniature marshmallows

½ C chopped pecans

Beat egg yolks; add vinegar, sugar, butter and seasonings. Mix well. Cook over low heat for about 3 minutes. Remove from heat, cool. Whip cream when ready to serve. Fold in whipped cream, marshmallows and nuts into the cooled mixture. Wonderful for fruit salads.

Pickling Recipes

Quick Fresh-Pack Whole Dill Pickles:
8 pounds of pickling cucumbers (3–5 inch)
1 1/4 C canning or pickling salt
2 gallons cold water
1 ½ quarts cider vinegar
1/4 C sugar
2 quarts water
2 T whole mixed pickling spices
5 T whole mustard seeds
21 heads of fresh dill or 7 T dill seed
Yield: 7 quarts or 14 pints.

Wash cucumbers. Cut 1/16 inch slice from blossom end and discard. Leave 1/4 inch of stem attached. Dissolve 3/4 C salt in 2 gallons of water. Pour over cucumbers and let stand 12 hours. Drain.

Combine cider vinegar, ½ C salt, sugar and 2 quarts of water. Add mixed pickling spices tied in a clean white cloth. Heat to boiling.

Fill jars with cucumbers. Add 2 tsp mustard seed and 3 heads of fresh dill to each quart. Use half the amount for pints. Cover with boiling pickling solution, leaving ½ inch headspace. Remove air bubbles. Wipe jar rims. Adjust lids.

Process in a boiling water bath: pints—15 minutes at 6,000 feet or less, 20 minutes above 6,000 feet; quarts—20 minutes at

6,000 feet or below, 25 minutes above 6,000 feet (Kendall 1989.)

Quick Sweet Pickles:
8 pounds of 3 to 4 inch pickling cucumbers
1/3 C canning or pickling salt
Crushed or cubed ice
4 ½ C sugar
3 ½ C cider vinegar
2 tsp celery seeds
1 T whole allspice
2 T mustard seed
Yield: 7 to 9 pints.

Wash cucumbers. Cut 1/16 inch off the blossom end and discard. Cut cucumbers into slices or strips. Place in large bowl and sprinkle with 1/3 C salt. Cover with 2 inches of crushed or cubed ice. Refrigerate 3 to 4 hours. Add more ice as needed.

Combine sugar, cider vinegar, celery seeds, allspice and mustard seed in a 3 quart sauce pot. Heat to boiling.

Drain cucumbers and pack without heating into clean jars, leaving ½ inch headspace. Fill jars to ½ inch from top with hot liquid. Remove air bubbles with a plastic spatula. Wipe jar rims. Adjust lids.

Process in a boiling water bath for the same amount of time as indicated in the Quick Fresh-Pack Whole Dill Pickles recipe. After processing and cooling, store jars 4 to 5 weeks before opening to allow for flavor development. Add 2 slices of raw onion to each jar before filling, if desired (Kendall 1989).

> <u>Pickled Sweet Green Tomatoes:</u>
> 10 to 11 pounds of green tomatoes (16 cups sliced 1/4 inch thick)
> 2 C thinly sliced onions
> 1/4 C canning or pickling salt
> 3 C brown sugar
> 4 C cider vinegar
> 1 T each of mustard seed, allspice, celery seed and whole cloves
> Yield: 9 pints or 4 ½ quarts.

Wash and slice tomatoes and onions. Place in bowl, sprinkle with 1/4 C salt and let stand 4 to 6 hours. Drain.

Heat and stir sugar in vinegar until dissolved. Tie mustard seed, allspice, celery seed and cloves in a spice bag. Add to cider vinegar with tomatoes and onions. If needed, add minimum water to cover pieces. Bring to a boil and simmer 30 minutes, stirring as needed to prevent burning. Tomatoes should be tender and transparent when properly cooked. Remove spice bag.

Fill jars and cover with hot pickling solution, leaving ½ inch headspace. Remove air bubbles. Wipe jar rims and adjust lids.

Process in a boiling water bath: pints—15 minutes at 6,000 feet or below, 20 minutes above 6,000 feet; quarts—20 minutes at 6,000 feet or below, 25 minutes above 6,000 feet (Kendall 1989).

Reduced-sodium Sliced Sweet Dill Pickles:
4 pounds pickling cucumbers
6 C cider vinegar
6 C sugar
2 T canning or pickling salt
1 ½ tsp celery seed
1 ½ tsp mustard seed
2 large onions, thinly sliced
8 heads fresh dill
Yield: About 8 pints.

Wash cucumbers. Cut off the blossom end and discard. Cut cucumbers into 1/4 inch slices. Combine cider vinegar, sugar, salt, celery and mustard seeds in a large saucepan. Bring this mixture to a boil. Place 2 slices of onion and 1 dill head in each pint jar. Fill jars with cucumber slices, leaving ½ inch space from the rim. Add 1 slice of onion and 1 dill head on top. Pour hot pickling solution over cucumbers, leaving 1/4 inch headspace. Remove air bubbles; wipe jar rims and adjust lids. Process in a boiling water bath according to prior pickling recipes recommendations.

Remove jars from canner and cool upright on a rack or towel overnight. Label and store in a cool, dark, dry place (Kendall 1989).

CLEANING

Cider vinegar can be used for many different cleaning jobs around the house. I will list in alphabetical order some of the jobs and give a few details on the amount to use, other solutions to add and procedures to follow:

Aluminum discoloration

1 T cider vinegar to 1 cup of water. Boil the vinegar and place the discolored utensils in the solution until they are clean. It may take more than one treatment.

Bath tub film

Wipe tub with cider vinegar and then baking soda and rinse.

Brick fix

Clean fireplace bricks with a mixture of equal parts vinegar, borax and ammonia. Your bricks will shine.

Carpet renewal

After cleaning the carpet, add 1 cup of cider vinegar to your rinse water. This will help take out any remaining soap residue left in the carpet. It will help to keep your carpet cleaner longer as soap residue attracts dirt.

Carpet stain removal

Add 1 tsp of cider vinegar to a pint of warm water and 1 tsp of liquid detergent. Keep this mixture in a closed jar and use when spills occur.

Clothes washing

Add 1 cup of cider vinegar to the last rinse cycle. It dissolves the alkalines in soaps and detergents.

Cutting grease

A few teaspoons of cider vinegar will help cut through grease.

Furniture Polish

Make your own furniture polish by mixing one part cider vinegar and three parts olive oil and use a soft cloth.

Garbage disposal cleaner

Make cider vinegar ice cubes. Put one cup of vinegar in a solution of water and fill your ice trays. Freeze. Run the frozen cubes through the disposal and then flush with cold water for a few minutes.

Shining Formica counters

Clean with a soft cloth soaked in cider vinegar.

Stain removal (Crawford 1988)

Beer: Soak in cider vinegar solution, flush with water, sponge with alcohol, wash and use chlorine bleach if safe for the fabric.

Black coffee: Soak in vinegar, flush with water, sponge with alcohol, wash and bleach.

Dye which is not red or yellow: Soak in vinegar, flush, dry completely, sponge with alcohol, dry completely, soak in ammonia solution, flush with water, wash with a chlorine bleach, if safe for the fabric.

Fruit and fruit juices: Soak in vinegar, flush in water, sponge with alcohol, wash and use chlorine bleach if safe.

White glue: Sponge with water, soak in a vinegar solution, sponge with alcohol and wash.

Jelly or jam: Soak in cider vinegar, rinse, sponge with alcohol, wash and bleach.

Liquor: Follow the same procedure as for Jelly.

Perspiration: Soak in ammonia solution, rinse, soak in a vinegar solution, rinse, dry completely, sponge with alcohol, wash with chlorine bleach, if safe for fabric.

Red dye and ink: Follow the same procedure as for perspiration.

Suntan lotion: Soak in a vinegar solution, rinse, sponge with alcohol, wash and bleach.

Tannin stain: Absorb any excess liquid creating the stain; try not to force the stain into the fabric. Use a cider vinegar solution on the stain.

Tea: Follow the same procedure as for Suntan lotion.

Urine: Soak in ammonia solution, rinse, soak in vinegar, rinse, dry completely, sponge with alcohol, wash and bleach.

Wine: Follow the same procedure as for Suntan lotion.

When the word solution is mentioned here, use the following:

Vinegar: 1 quart warm water, ½ tsp liquid dishwashing detergent, 1 T cider vinegar.

Ammonia: 1 quart warm water, ½ tsp liquid dishwashing detergent, 1 T ammonia.

Bleach: 1 tsp chlorine bleach, 1 tsp water.

Tea Kettle deposits

Boil ½ cup of cider vinegar in the tea kettle which is filled with water.

Toilet bowl cleaner

Deodorize the toilet bowl with 3 cups of cider vinegar. Allow the vinegar to remain in the water for at least ½ hour and then flush.

Washing woodwork, windows, wood paneling

Cider vinegar in a solution of water is excellent for general cleaning of woodwork, windows and wood paneling. It is also used on the walls and floors of yachts which have been to sea to remove the oily residue left by sea spray (Diggs 1989).

COSMETIC

For your skin to be healthy, free from dry patches and rashes, it needs a slightly acid mantle. When your skin has an alkaline mantle, it will be dry, cracked and itchy. You might want to check your urine with testing paper to determine if your system is alkaline in general.

Bathing in warm water with cider vinegar or using a diluted solution as an after-bath splash can help maintain the correct body chemistry and protect against dry, flaky skin. A few drops of cosmetic vinegar in a basin of water gives you a facial bath that can tone and freshen your skin marvelously. You can make twenty-four ounces at home for about five dollars. You can save money making your own cosmetics.

The following is a suggested recipe for a cider vinegar cosmetic solution. Take two ounces each of the fresh herbs listed here or once ounce if they are dried. Place the herbs in a stone or glass jar.

Bruise them thoroughly and then add a quart of boiling vinegar. Cover the jar tightly and let it stand in a warm place. Shake the contents occasionally so as to disturb the mixture. After two weeks strain off the clear liquid vinegar. In a different bottle combine 1/4 ounce gum camphor, ½ ounce gum benzoin and 3/4 T of alcohol–at least 75 percent proof. When these ingredients are dissolved, add the vinegar mixture. Let his mixture stand for three days and then filter the liquid through fine linen or clean blotting paper or a coffee filter. Bottle, cork and seal this fragrant vinegar and use as described above.

Use cider vinegar to restore the skin's natural acid balance. Combine one small handful each of: orange flowers, orange peel, orange leaves, rose leaves, rose buds, rose hips, white willow bark and camomile. Pour one quart of boiling vinegar over this mixture. Let it steep in a closed glass container, shaking the container daily, until the materials have lost their color. Strain. Add one cup of rose water which you can obtain from a pharmacy or health food store. Let settle for one week. Open, strain again and discard any sediment, saving the remaining liquid. This is a most wonderful astringent, body wash or hair rinse. Be careful with rinsing hair which has been permed because vinegar may shorten the life of the perm. This solution is good for the scalp and hair in general–just not so good for perms.

Rose Vinegar

Steep one ounce rose petals and one handful camomile flowers in two cups of cider vinegar for one week. Strain and add one cup of rose water to the liquid. Dip a soft cloth in the rose vinegar and use it as an astringent wash for the face or body.

Botanical Cider Vinegars

To make a facial vinegar, soak one ounce of the botanicals (flowers and herbs) of your choice in two cups of cider vinegar. You can use acacia flowers, clover, orange, elder flowers for dry skin; cucumber, lemon, witch hazel or lemon grass for oily skin; or rose buds, camomile flowers or mints for normal skin. Steep for two weeks, shaking daily. Strain. Let it settle for a few days and then pour off the clear, colorful cider vinegar. To use, dilute the vinegar with a little rose water, orange flower water or just plain water. Splash it on your face or body or rub it into the roots of your hair. Be careful not to get the vinegar solution in or near your eyes.

HOUSEHOLD HELPERS AND OTHERS

Ant deterrent

Wash counter tops, cabinets and floors with a warm solution of 1 cup of cider vinegar to a gallon of water.

Blanket renewal

Add 2 cups of cider vinegar to the rinse cycle when you next wash a blanket.

Cane chair rejuvenation

Sponge a hot solution of half-vinegar-half-water onto any cane chair with sagging seats. Place the chair in the sun to dry. This will renew your cane chair.

Clogged drain

Pour a handful of baking soda into the drain. Add half a cup of cider vinegar and let it work for about an hour before running any water. This solution will cut through soap scum and minor accumulations in the drain trap.

Cold hands

The next time you need to work outside on a very cold day, rinse your hands in vinegar and then dry them before going out. The vinegar wash makes the frigid temperatures easier to take and seems to keep the fingers limber a little longer.

Cut-flower preservation

Add 2 T of cider vinegar and 3 T of sugar to a quart of warm water.

Decal removal

Sponge on cider vinegar, wait a few minutes and then wash off.

Deodorant

The acidity of the skin provides some protection against bacterial invasion. Dab underarms daily with straight vinegar. Let it dry on the skin without rinsing while you towel off the rest of your body. You will have no more problem with perspiration odor.

Galvanized-finish remover

If you want to paint a galvanized-finished roof or other items, you will need to remove the galvanized finish before painting in order for the paint to adhere. Wash the area you want to paint with straight cider vinegar and then rinse thoroughly. This removes the finish beautifully and the paint you apply will now adhere.

Grass Killer

Pour undiluted cider vinegar directly on the grass growing between the cracks in your sidewalks or any other place you do not want the grass or weeds to grow.

Lime fighter

Neutralize the harsh, drying effects of garden lime by dousing your hands freely with vinegar. Rinse with cold water.

No-frost windshield

Wipe on a solution of 3 parts vinegar to 1 part water.

Paint brush softener

Soak the hard brush in hot vinegar and then wash with warm soapy water and rinse once again with vinegar and water solution. Then just rinse with water and let dry.

Plaster

If you want your wet plaster to take longer to set up, mix a half teaspoon of cider vinegar into each quart of plaster. This will give you more working time.

Propane lanterns

For longer-lasting and brighter-burning wicks, soak new wicks for several hours in vinegar and then let them dry before inserting.

Renew shoes

To remove salt stains, pour vinegar on a damp cloth and wipe the affected areas. Then polish with a soft cloth (Heinz 1989).

Room odors

Place a small bowl of cider vinegar with your favorite herbs or dried flowers in the warmest corner of your home. This will remove the smell of fresh paint and stale tobacco.

Rust cutter

Soak the rusted bolt or nut with undiluted cider vinegar. You may want to use a small brush, and it may take a number of applications. If you have the time, let it work overnight.

Tarnished brass or copper

Mix salt, flour and vinegar into a paste. Apply the paste to the tarnished item and leave on for about an hour. Then rub it off with a soft cloth and wash.

CHAPTER 6

METHODS OF MAKING CIDER VINEGAR

There have been many methods for making cider vinegar. The excellence to which cider vinegar can reach through scientific methods, great care and much time—either in the home or in commercial production—is an interesting story. To acquire perspective and understanding as to why cider vinegar is processed as it is today, we will start with early methods. In the following pages you will note that the primary emphasis is on the initial cider production. Before you can make vinegar, you must make cider.

EARLY METHODS

The best cider was made by New England farmers, using their own apples and their own hand-built cider presses. People argued about which apples were the best for cider. To these farmers making cider from rotten, dirty, wormy apples which had fallen to the ground was an insult to the art of cider making. Perfectionists felt that all apples should be examined and blemishes cut out, washed and wiped dry. Apples were cored, and the chief reason for removing the core before making cider was to avoid crushing the apple seeds which would leave a bitter taste in the juice (Orton 1973).

Cider making was a family affair. There were superstitions pertaining to its making, especially about the weather. The best cider was made when the wind blew from the west or northwest. Cider would have an unpleasant taste if made when the wind was blowing from the south.

During the 19th century there were numerous recipes for blending apples to make good cider. The flavor of the cider was the main reason for blending apples. Apples were selected for their high sugar and acid content. Both these properties were determined by tasting the apples rather than by scientific tests. The early farmers managed to arrive at a good balance between acidity and sweetness just by taste.

There is a wide range of tastes in apples, and they can vary from 6 percent to 20 percent in sugar and in acid from 1/10 of 1 percent to over 1 percent. Considering this wide variation, it is highly possible that the taste test used by these New England farmers was a pretty good test for choosing apples. Generally, a farmer used the apples from his own farm.

After the apples were selected and washed, they were ground or mashed into a pulp called pomace. This was like coarse, uncooked applesauce with skins. A stone wheel was used to mash the apples. It was similar to the old stone grinding mill used to grind grain. The wheel was turned by real horse power. Seeds and peels were in this pulp, that is, unless you were one of the perfectionists who removed the cores. Most farmers felt that the seeds did no harm because the pressing did not crush them. Grinding the apples into a pulp was usually done at night. The mash was then left to stand which gave it a darker color which we understand today as an oxidation process.

The cider press was a simple machine, usually made by the farmer himself from hand-hewn ten-inch beams and a massive wood screw. Some presses had one screw; others had two. At the bottom of each screw was an opening for inserting a stout pole or lever. The threaded top part of each screw turned inside a threaded hole in the big cross beam of the frame.

Turning these massive screws was often done manually. Those who had horses used horse power. The pressure exerted on the apple pomace from the top by a series of pressboards produced the cider juice which trickled down into a channel and then into an open tub. This was sweet cider. This pressing was repeated until the last drop of cider was obtained and then the pomace was given to the pigs–nothing was wasted. The methods of extracting juice varied over the centuries but the general principle remained the same–to get all the juice out of all the apples.

Besides much argumentation about what apples to blend, farmers argued about fermentation processes. The simple way was to take the sweet cider as it came from the press into the tub, pour it at once into clean wooden barrels or casks and then carefully regulate the vent. If the vent was too small, fermentation from the natural yeast in the air would burst open the barrel. Much care was taken so fermentation would be a long, slow affair. The slower the process the better the cider.

Some people were not satisfied with this natural, unhurried, unprocessed method. They added yeast, sugar, raisins, spices, saltpeter, alum to help regulate the process and improve the flavor.

The next step in the process was to put the juice into clean casks several times. This was called *racking*. It was a form of filtering as sediment settled to the bottom. White bubbles would appear on the surface of the solution. As soon as the bubbles appeared, it was time to rack again. When the fermentation finally ceased after several rackings, the cider was poured into clean barrels. The decision as to how many rackings cider needed was a matter of experience and taste. When the cider liquid was fairly clear and bright, and no hissing sound could be heard, or there was not enough internal air pressure to blow out a candle flame held to the bunghole, the farmer would stop the fermentation process.

The earliest method of making vinegar from alcoholic cider was to just expose it to air and let it age. The first recognized method to produce vinegar would be the slow process, also known as the Orleans process.

The Orleans process used a barrel of about 50 gallon capacity. The alcoholic liquid apple cider was poured into the barrel, and a small amount of vinegar containing a mass of vinegar bacteria, mother of vinegar, was added to start the reaction. One or two small air holes were drilled above the liquid level to expose the surface to aeration. The finished vinegar was drawn off through a wooden spigot near the bottom of the barrel. Care was taken in refilling the barrel with new alcoholic cider to avoid breaking up the surface film of bacteria. The mixture of vinegar and alcoholic cider was allowed to remain in the barrel until its maximum acid content developed—up to three months. Then, two-thirds to three-fourths of the vinegar was withdrawn and replaced with fresh alcoholic cider and the process repeated.

MODERN METHODS

Modern methods still start with apples selected for condition, maturity and variety. Sound, firm apples are best. Sound apples have no bruises, worms or rotten patches. They are washed to remove foreign matter and dirt.

Walter H. Hildrick, Jr., of Sterling Cider Company, one of New England's oldest commercial producers of cider products said, "The primary requirement for the good juice is to start off with good, sound fruit, thoroughly washed and rinsed clean, unpolluted water and then promptly pressed, filtered and bottled in a sanitary manner. New England has long been noted for its fine-flavored apples. More apples are grown in the state of Washington than in any other state, and they are beautiful. But for flavor, New England fruit is superior. We were informed by a leading orchardist years ago that the primary reason for this is the soil of New England is made up of glacial deposits left here many centuries ago, rich in minerals and trace elements, which make the fruit healthful and so flavorful. The soil on the West Coast, however, consists largely of volcanic ash and seems to lack something New England soil has."

Authorities agree that a blend of apples makes a fine cider with a finer balance of sweetness, tang, aroma and body. Three or more varieties of apples are preferred to one. How to choose the varieties to blend is an old question. It basically depends on individual taste.

The U.S. Department of Agriculture (USDA) can provide current bulletins on the subject of cider making. You can write for their bulletins by addressing your inquiry to: U.S. Department of Agriculture, 14th Street and Independence Avenue S.W., Washington, D.C. 20250. You can also contact them online by going to www.usda.gov.

For convenience purposes, the USDA has divided apples into four groups: (1) Sweet—Beauty, Stark, Delicious, Grimes, Cortland; (2) Mildly acid to slightly tart—Winesap, Jonathan, Stayman, Northern Spy, York, Imperial, Wealthy, Rhode Island Greening, Newton-Pippin ; (3) Aromatic—Golden Delicious, Winter Banana, Ribston, Transcendent, Martha; (4) Crab apples—very astringent, highly acid and rich in tannin. Tannin has an antiseptic influence on the bacteria which cause bad cider. A little tannin acts as an inhibitor of enzymes and makes cider keep longer and better. Only small amounts of crab apples should be used in a blend.

No two cider makers will agree on how to create the best blend. They do agree that apples should be blended. The general rule applied is 1/3 tart (late-fall or winter apples) and 2/3 sweet (mid-fall apples).

After the apples have been selected and washed, the process of making pomace is next. Modern methods use power machines–a grater and a hammer mill. There are two types of cider presses today. One is the mechanical device that presses using heavy threaded screws. The other operates with a hydraulic ram which forces down the top and several pressboards to exert pressure on the pomace placed in the machine. The screened juice is collected in receiving tanks and then pumped into storage tanks for fermentation into alcohol.

The process of changing alcohol into acetic acid has been speeded up. The two more advanced methods of this process are known as the generator process and the submerged process.

The generator process, first introduced into Germany, has been used almost universally for over 100 years for the production of commercial vinegars. A typical generator is a cylindrical wooden tank equipped with cooling coils, air vents and a grating two or more feet above the bottom to support packing material, preferably beechwood shavings, and a sparger for dispersal of vinegar stock evenly over the surface of the packing. The liquid trickles over the packing which is covered with vinegar bacteria, mother of vinegar, and meets a rising current of air admitted through the bottom. Circulation is continued until acetification is practically complete.

The submerged process for making vinegar is an outgrowth of the spectacular technological advances made in antibiotic manufacture during World War II. The submerged method employs a cylindrical stainless steel or wood tank suitably equipped with devices for ensuring an adequate, continuous air supply and cooling coils to control temperature fluctuations. To start acetification, the unit is filled with a mixture of vinegar containing bacteria, mother of vinegar, and the alcoholic cider to be oxidized, supplemented with nutrients and aerated. The temperature is maintained at about 86 degrees F. After acetification about half of the vinegar is withdrawn and the remainder is left in the tank as seed or mother for the next batch. This method, in one form or another, developed in West Germany and the United States, is rapidly replacing the older processes throughout the world (The Encyclopedia Americana 1980).

Once in the bottle, it is important that the vinegar does not oxidize or grow molds. It is, therefore, necessary to add substances which deter the oxygen from affecting the vinegar. The usual substance is sulphur dioxide. Some producers use vitamin C. There are other problems that arise from speeding up the process such as polyphenol hazes, and these problems will be discussed in greater detail in the chapter on Commercial Production.

COMMERCIAL PRODUCTION OF CIDER VINEGAR

In the United States there is a substantial processed-apple industry which generates a considerable amount of peels and cores as apple waste. Up to 50 percent of the apple juice used in cider production may come from pressings of this material, as well as from fresh juice. Pectolytic enzymes or hot-water leaching may be utilized on the waste before it is passed to the mill and press to increase the juice yield. A disadvantage associated with the extraction of juice from peels and cores is that the content of non-sugar solids increases, particularly the procyanidin polyphenols which are concentrated in these regions of the fruit. This may cause problems at a later stage.

The juice mixture, from fresh or concentrated sources plus the pressings from peels and cores, is pumped into fermentation tanks where a natural yeast fermentation is usually allowed to work. Some plants inoculate the juice with a specific yeast. This fermentation to an alcohol content of from 5 to 6 percent usually takes only a week or so. Yeast fermentations are generally not temperature controlled. Nutrients are not normally added to the fermentation mixture, except in the case where the juice was entirely from concentrate. Ammonium phosphate and thiamin may be added to concentrates, which are often lacking in amino nitrogen and B vitamins essential for yeast growth. After fermentation, the cider is allowed to age for at least a month before moving to the acetification process.

Acetification

The half-filled barrel process (Orleans) and the packed-generator process (Quick) have been replaced with the continuously aerated submerged-culture fermenters. It is recognized that there are two genera of acetic acid bacteria: The Gluconobacter and the Acetobacter. Only the Acetobacter are used for vinegar production. In actual practice, most vinegar producers probably do not select particular bacterial strains. Rather, fermentation conditions are experimentally optimized and whatever bacteria in the solution and air that proliferate under the optimized conditions are "selected" for the fermentation.

A submerged-culture fermenter has a vortex stirrer mounted at the base of the fermenter tank which sucks in air and distributes it continuously to the cider and Acetobacter mixture. Bacterial growth is rapid. A foam breaker is located in the head of the tank for continual foam removal. When the fermenter is operated properly, the withdrawal of the finished product and addition of fresh cider can be repeated indefinitely.

The conversion of alcohol to acetic acid is monitored by an alkograph. This system can automatically discharge vinegar and take in fresh cider when the alcohol level in the fermenter falls below 0.1 to 0.2 percent. The advantage of this system over the older systems is that it will convert the cider more rapidly than the older types. They may be operated on a continuous or semi-continuous basis with little need for regular cleaning. They are almost entirely free of A. xylinum. They do, however, require a constant supply of air. Even a one-minute cessation in the air supply is sufficient to kill most of the Acetobacter cells in submerged-culture units. Temperature control to within a degree or so is also extremely important. They are operated at between 30–35 degrees C., which requires a cooling water flow under normal conditions. The organisms may die if the cooling system fails. The presence of sulfur dioxide or other contaminants in the air supply may also have an inhibitory effect on the Acetobacter.

Overall, the advantages of submerged-culture systems outweigh their disadvantages. They are now standard for cider vinegar production. In most plants, the cider stock is fortified with nutrients before acetification, i.e. ammonium carbonate, ammonium sulfate and ammonium monophosphate (Lea 1989).

Maturation

After acetification is completed, the vinegar is pumped into wooden or stainless-steel tanks for storage and maturation. In some plants it may undergo a rough filtration at this stage. In the past, maturation was considered desirable for development of flavor, for clarification and for reduction of postbottling haze. Maturation for close to a year was usual until recently. With increased production demands and the cost of storage capacity, cider vinegar is often matured now for only a month or two at best.

Clarification

Practices vary widely. In the basic, standard procedure, vinegar is rough-filtered, diluted with water to the required acidic strength for retail sale (5 percent), passed through a plate heat exchanger for pasteurization at 65 to 85 degrees C., and hot-filled into glass bottles or cooled before cold filling into plastic bottles or flasks. A high pasteurization temperature is recommended for vinegars from submerged-culture fermenters because this vinegar contains many more Acetobacter than traditional vinegars.

Many variations on this standard procedure are possible. If a cider vinegar is not well-aged, it may be treated with activated carbon or with Polyclar AT (polyvinyl polypyrrolidore) after rough filtration and before dilution. This is done to absorb and remove the polyphenols which are responsible for post-bottle hazes. An alternative to rough filtration is *fining*, a process of adding substances that will collect the suspended materials and then settle to the bottom of the container. Fining reduces the total load of suspended material, principally Acetobacter, and may help to reduce the haze contributing polyphenols. A typical fining procedure is the addition of isinglass or gelatin followed by a slurry of bentonite. The mixture is stirred well and then left to settle for at least a week before racking. A quicker and easier method is the use of kieselsol, a form of silicon dioxide, followed by gelatin which forms compact bottoms within hours. The optimal amount of fining agent will vary from batch to batch. Fining generally does not result in a totally bright product. It does considerably lessen the load of subsequent filtration steps by removing the majority of the suspended material and it helps to reduce the occurrence of postbottling haze.

Bottling

In some cases the pasteurization step is replaced by cold sterile bottling through a microporous membrane. The purpose of pasteurization is to kill the remaining Acetobacter so that the acetification process does not continue in the bottle and form a mother of vinegar. In the old sterile process there is still the chance that Acetobacters can get in. If oxygen permeates the seal and the heat rises, there can be a problem. Pasteurization is the only effective procedure for killing the remaining bacteria.

Elimination of oxygen is also important in preventing postbottling haze formation from non-microbiological causes. Vinegars in polyethylene bottles, which are generally air-permeable, tend to be more susceptible to postbottling haze formation than those in glass. Polyvinylchloride containers are becoming more popular.

Additives

Various agents have been added to cider vinegar at the bottling stage, mostly to prevent excessive haze formation. The most effective of these agents is undoubtedly sulfur dioxide. Its effectiveness arises from its antimicrobial properties, which are enhanced by the low pH, and from its antioxidant, enzyme-inhibiting, and carbonyl-binding functions, which effectively block all modes of polyphenol polymerization.

Ascorbic acid (vitamin C) is considerably less effective unless used in very high dosages since it is only an antioxidant. Unfortunately, its breakdown products are carbonyls, which are potent pro-oxidants and will encourage haze formation. The addition of small amounts of ascorbic acid to cider vinegar is probably worse than useless. Pectin and gum arabic have also been added to cider vinegar to stabilize it against haze formation (Lea 1989).

Ultrafiltration

To avoid the use of additives and the problems associated with them, ultrafiltration has recently been promoted as an alternative method of stabilizing cider vinegars. In this technique the raw vinegar is pumped continuously and partly recirculated past membranes with typical cutoff of 50,000 molecular weight. The result is clarified cider vinegar. All yeasts, bacteria, and high-molecular-weight compounds are retained in the recirculating feed. In theory this technique should result in a completely stable cider vinegar.

Ultrafiltration is considered a help in removing acetification debris and Acetobacters. Filtration and sterilization may be done in one continuous operation. This should be done immediately before bottling. If vinegar is diluted with water, the product is flash-pasteurized at bottling time.

Despite its advantages, ultrafiltration will not always prevent haze. The haze-precursor molecules can easily pass through the smallest of ultrafiltration membranes and form hazes later.

Flow chart for cider vinegar production

The following flow chart will give you a graphic idea of the processing stages and addition of additives.

FLOW CHART

DELIVERY OF APPLES TO FACTORY
PRESSES EXTRACT APPLE JUICE
TRANSFERRED TO TANKS FOR ALCOHOLIC FERMENTATION
ROUGH FILTRATION/FINING
TRANSFERRED TO TANKS FOR ACETIFICATION
FILTRATION
AGED AND MATURED
REDUCE VINEGAR TO 5% ACIDITY
FILTERED/FINING
PASTEURIZATION
FILL AND CAP BOTTLES
LABEL AND CODE
SHIP

Defects and Problems

The major problems encountered in the production of cider vinegar are mother-of-vinegar growth, non-microbiological hazes occurring before and after bottling and vinegar eels.

Mother of Vinegar

Mother of vinegar, Acetobacter xylinum or A. xylinum for short, is essentially the vinegar-generating organism in the barrel process. It is distinguished from Acetobacter aceti (A.

aceti) by its ability to secrete sheets of cellulose. These cellulose sheets had the advantage of keeping the organisms afloat and in contact with air in the barrel process. In some of the more modern methods of production, the slimy cellulose material can coat the equipment impeding the flow of both air and liquid.

A. aceti inoculated into the acetification fermentation process may mutate to A. xylinum and cellulose production will gradually increase. At acid levels above 8 percent, A. xylinum seems to be inhibited.

Submerged-culture fermenters, when originally inoculated with strains of A. aceti, do not seem to produce A. xylinum even at low acid levels of about 5 percent, and so this problem does not arise. This is a distinct advantage to submerged-culture fermenters for cider vinegar production. If A. xylinum persists through the bottle product, due to a failure in pasteurization for instance, and if air can enter through a poorly sealed cap, it makes for a typical growth (Lea 1989).

Polyphenol Hazes

Biological problems such as vinegar eels and mother of vinegar are relatively easy to identify and to eliminate by pasteurization. It is more difficult to combat non-microbiological hazes and sediments that develop slowly in bottle storage. Such problems are often attributed to protein, but this belief is erroneous. In cider vinegar polyphenols are likely to be the chief cause of hazes. Apple juices and cider vinegars are relatively deficient in protein but contain larger quantities of polyphenols than do white wines or beers.

The four major classes of polyphenols in apples are phenolic acids, dihydrochalcones, catechins and procyanidins. The procyanidins, formerly known as leucocyanidins or simply as tannins, are oligomers. They are the most important polyphenolic haze precursors because of their susceptibility to further polymerization. There are three mechanisms which contribute to further polymerization. The first one is pH dependent and proceeds more rapidly at lower ph. Mechanism (2) and (3) are oxygen and carbonyl dependent. **All three mechanisms can be blocked by sulfur dioxide**, which explains why it has been used as a vinegar stabilizer. Mechanism (1) will proceed in cider vinegar even in the absence of oxygen, and so a cider vinegar is potentially unstable as long as any procyanidins remain (Lea 1989).

During the long traditional aging of cider vinegar, most of the procyanidins polymerize, both oxidatively and otherwise, eventually settled to the bottom of the container. Thus, the product was relatively stable when bottled. If vinegar is not so aged, the procyanidins continue to polymerize non-oxidatively in the bottle and produce a haze.

If sulfur dioxide is not used as a preservative, it is important to reduce the content of procyanidins as well as the level of oxygen in the bottle. Procyanidin reduction can be achieved either by long aging or by a fining agent with an affinity for procyanidins (such as gelatin/kieselsol or gelatin/bentonite). Further procyanidin reduction may be achieved by treating with activated charcoal or by constant stirring of the vinegar with Polyclar AF. Following such treatment, the vinegar must be bottled immediately with minimum contact with oxygen.

By a combination of these techniques, it is possible to produce cider vinegar that is stable for many months in the bottle without the use of preservatives.

A quick assessment of the procyanidin content may be made by mixing equal parts of 50 percent HCI and 10 percent formaldehyde solution with clarified cider vinegar. If a detectable haze does not form within one hour, the vinegar may be regarded as low in procyanidins and relatively stable. The amount of procyanidin is relative to the original source of the apple juice. **Peels and cores have a high procyanidin content** (Lea 1989).

Vinegar Eels

Vinegar eels, nematodes of the species Anguillula aceti, are carried by fruit flies. They live at the top of fermentation and storage vessels, independent of light and oxygen. They may appear at any stage in the production of vinegar. They are less common in submerged-culture fermenters than in the old-style packed generators and are chiefly found during the storage and maturation of vinegar, particularly in wooden vats.

As yet, it has not been determined if they are beneficial or harmful. Some believe that the eels scavenge dead Acetobacter and keep the acetification active. Others believe that the eels are harmful because they reduce the total bacterial count and lower the final acidity of the vinegar. Most of the time their affect on the vinegar itself is insignificant.

Since the eels are removed by filtration and both they and their eggs are killed by pasteurization, they do not present a problem to the consumer. Good hygiene can reduce the number of eels within and around a factory (Lea 1989).

DO-IT-YOURSELF HOME PRODUCTION OF CIDER VINEGAR

You should by now have some perspective on how apple cider vinegar was and is made. It is not a simple matter of combining peels, cores and bruised apples, left after making applesauce, in a crock or jar and covering with water. You will not get apple cider vinegar. You will get, most likely, a smelly mess. If you want to make your own cider vinegar, it will take some time and effort.

Reasons Why You Might Want to Make Your Own

Because the process is time consuming and takes some effort, you might want to first check out the available brands in your stores. If you have any questions as to the quality, type of apples, additives, etc., write to the producer. If you are not satisfied with what is available at the market, then consider producing your own.

If you are considering using apple cider vinegar as a medicinal remedy or using it on a regular basis in your diet, you will certainly want to feel confident in the quality of the particular cider vinegar you are using. If you make your own, then you know for certain how it was processed, filtered, aged and the quality of apples used. Remember, commercial production adds substances and pasteurizes because they don't have the time to age.

Another reason why you might want to make your own is that there are many different kinds and qualities of vinegars. We discussed imitation and synthetic vinegars in an earlier chapter. Distilled vinegar is a vinegar which has been heated to turn it to steam and then distilled. This process destroys enzymes and distills out minerals such as potassium, phosphorus, chlorine, natural organic sodium, magnesium, sulphur, iron, copper, natural organic fluorine, silicon and many other trace minerals. It also destroys the natural malic acid which is very important in fighting body toxins. This vinegar is made directly from acetous fermentation of distilled ethyl alcohol after the addition of nutrient salts.

After considering the brands on the market, the various kinds of vinegar, and the purpose for which you want to use your cider vinegar, you might decide you are ready for a new hobby. Homemade apple cider vinegar will also make wonderful gifts for friends and family who care about their health. So, let's get started!

How to Get Started—Your Work Space

First, look around your house, apartment, condo or garage for a space–a work space. The space must be an area that can be kept extremely clean, have some method of temperature control and adequate storage space for aging. You may want two spaces–one for production and another for aging and storing. Most bacteria are sensitive to ultraviolet light. Fermentation will proceed faster in a place void of light. During the fermentation process put the cider in a dark area–total darkness is desirable. The bacteria do need a source of oxygen. The more oxygen provided, the faster the rate of production of the bacteria and your product. Oxygen can come right from the air but it must be readily available.

Your aging container should be stationary in your work space. Movement of the container will retard production. It may also cause the "mother" to fall to the bottom and rot. We are talking about the acetification process. A "fallen mother" will deteriorate the quality of your vinegar. If the vinegar is moved during the aging phase, the sediments will be stirred up again, causing a loss of one of the major benefits of aging.

Also take into consideration temperature control in your work space. Cider vinegar is produced at temperatures between 59-94 degrees F. and stored to age in a cool place, 40-50 degrees F.

When you have decided on the work space, you may want to make some alterations or build storage shelves before purchasing any equipment or making any vinegar.

Read and Talk

Gather as much reading material as you can on your new hobby and read until you have decided exactly how you want to proceed. Good sources of reading material are the Internet, your library, the U.S. Department of Agriculture bulletins and the bibliography in this book. Talk to any local supplier of equipment. Talk to anyone who is currently making their own cider vinegar.

Supplies and Equipment

When selecting or making your equipment, tools, utensils, keep in mind that only high-grade stainless steel can be used, particularly during the acetic acid production phase. Most other metals will react with the vinegar and ruin or poison it. Aluminum, copper, lead, zinc and iron are particularly dangerous. Wood, bamboo, ceramics, glass and enamel are materials you can use. Woods will add flavors and aromas to your vinegars. Bamboo, rubber, glass and plastics can be used for pipes and tubes. A clean coffee can with holes in the bottom can be used for the pressing of the apple juice if you use the homemade apple press illustrated in this chapter.

You will need:

1. Equipment to reduce your beautiful apples into a mash or pulp–knife, blender or food processor;

2. Equipment to press the juice from the pulp–homemade apple press or a cider/wine press which can be purchased from a local wine/beer-making supply shop. If you cannot

find any supplier in your local area or listed in your yellow pages, I suggest that you try the Internet. If you go to Google and type in Cider Press, a number of companies will come up such as: www.happyvalleyranch.com, www.MoreWineMaking.com, applejuicers.com, www.pleasanthillgrain.com, www.kuffelcreek.com, ciderpressreview.com, www.coldhollow.com, www.homesteadhelpers.com/fullciderpress.htm,; American Harvester makes a combination cider mill and press. They are located at Happy Valley Ranch, Paola, Kansas. Their double-tub allows both the grinding and squeezing to take place simultaneously. They say that two people can easily squeeze 50 gallons of cider in an afternoon with their equipment.

3. Cheesecloth for straining and covering containers;

4. White sheeting for pressing cloth;

5. A container for collecting the juice as it flows from the press;

6. A container for the first fermentation process of converting the sugar in the juice into alcohol. The size of your containers will depend on the volume you plan to make. To give you some idea, a bushel of apples should yield from 2 to 3 gallons of juice. Straight-sided stone jars holding from 4 to 6 gallons make excellent containers. Whisky or brandy barrels may be used. Vinegar barrels cannot be used during this process because the acetic acid remaining from the vinegar will prevent the growth of the yeast necessary for the first transformation of juice into

alcohol. New barrels, as well as all your equipment should be washed with scalding water;

7. Hydrometer to test the amount of sugar in the solution;*

8. Siphoning device for transferring the cider into other containers without disturbing the sediment at the bottom–purchase from supplier;

9. A container for the second fermentation process of converting alcohol into acetic acid. It should be another crock or barrel. In this case the container may be one that has previously contained good vinegar, for now is the time for the acetic-acid-forming bacteria to take over and convert the alcohol to vinegar;

10. Hydrometer to measure alcohol content;*

11. Substances if you want to do a fining process to your vinegar for appearance–purchase from supplies;

12. High-neck bottles, corks, wax and labels.

How to Build Your Own Home Cider Press

1. First start with determining the height of your base which will be made out of thick wood or bricks. You will want your base to be high enough to accommodate the container you want to use to collect the apple juice.

---

* There are several makes of hydrometers–Brix, Balling and Baume. Check with your equipment supplier for which hydrometer will meet all your needs. A good hydrometer should have instructions with it that will tell you the correct temperature at which it is to be used. You will need a good thermometer to take such test accurately.

2. You have your base ready. Cut 2 boards which are 8 inches wide and 1 inch thick 2 feet long. Drill 2 holes in one board to accept the dowels which will pass through when you press down on that board. We will call this board the top and the other the bottom board.

3. Drill or cut a 2 inch hole in the center of the bottom board to allow the juice pressed in the can to pass through.

4. Next, to the bottom board cut two holes which match the two holes in the top board. You may cut the two holes at the same time by placing one board on top of the other when the hole is cut. This will guarantee that both holes are identical.

5. Cut your two dowels the same length and long enough so that when there is pulp in the can and the top board is raised up, the top board is still on the dowels. The length of the dowels will depend upon the height of the container you use as the press container.

6. Glue or epoxy the two dowels into the holes in the bottom board and allow them to dry. Try to make certain that the dowels are straight while they are drying.

7. To the top board which has two holes in it on the sides, glue or epoxy the large dowel or board to the center underside and to that glue/epoxy the round piece of wood, which is the piece that presses on the pulp.

Now you have made your homemade apple press. You can add bricks or lead weights to help apply additional pressure when you press your pulp.

To press the pulp, line the container with clean sheeting cloth, fill with pulp to about 3 inches thick, cover the pulp with the excess edges of the cloth. This is considered a layer of pulp. You can press just one layer or make several other layers in the same manner.

Place the top board onto the dowels and begin to apply pressure. Apply pressure slowly to avoid rupturing the press cloths. Build up pressure, approximately 150 pounds per square inch, and hold for several minutes. Continue applying pressure throughout the day until you feel that all the juice is out of the pulp.

As you grow to understand the process, you will know what utensils and supplies to get. Power presses and other motor-driven equipment for producing large quantities of cider vinegar can also be purchased from a supplier—check the Internt (Orton 1973).

Clean, Clean and Clean

The quality and life of your cider in all its stages depends upon the cleanliness of the containers and of every single utensil or machine with which it comes in contact. The need to wash, scrub, clean and rinse cannot be too strongly emphasized. This includes the walls and ceilings of your work space. Cider is almost as volatile as milk. Never use soap or detergent to clean your equipment. Household bleach can be recommended but be certain to rinse away the bleach thoroughly. Use hot water.

The cleaner you keep your work space, the less problems you will have with fruit flies, vinegar mites and vinegar eels. Avoid vinegar spills and clean up spills and leaks immediately. These problems are covered in more detail at the end of this section of home production. The cleaner your work space, the better your cider will be.

Review of Basic Production Phases

Apples are washed, reduced to pulp and the juice is pressed out. The juice is put in containers to ferment into alcohol. The fermentation is caused by natural yeast in the air and yeast present on apple skins. Fermentation continues until the sugar in the juice has been converted to alcohol. This process takes about three to four weeks.

The next process is the making of acetic acid–vinegar. Acetification is the final process–the conversion of alcohol to acetic acid. Acetification is done by the Acetobacter bacteria. This bacteria converts carbohydrates into acetic acid. The more oxygen they have, the faster the acetification process. When this process is over, the cider vinegar is filtered and stored to develop flavor and remove sediment.

Technical Information

One part of sugar in apple juice should theoretically produce about 51 parts of alcohol. You will probably get more like 43 percent to 47 percent because some of the sugar is used by the yeast and other organisms for purposes other than alcohol production. In converting alcohol into acetic acid, 100 parts of alcohol should theoretically give 130 parts of acetic acid, but actually less than 120 parts are obtained because the bacteria and yeast use alcohol as food (Diggs 1989).

For every 100 parts of sugar in the apple juice, 50 to 55 parts of acetic acid should be produced. This means that if you want a cider vinegar containing about a 5 percent acetic acid, the fermentation should be started with at least a 10 percent sugar solution. The lower the acetic acid content you desire, the less sugar content in solution.

The Acetobacter will not grow well without certain inorganic salts such as potassium tartrate, ammonium phosphate and ammonium chloride. Yeast concentrations that have been properly sterilized seem to work well as Acetobacter nutrients.

Temperature control is most important. Cider vinegar is produced at temperatures between 59-94 degrees F. Temperatures below 59 degrees F. cause the production to fall too low. Above 94 degrees F. products begin to fail. The bacteria will die at 140 degrees F. Acetobacter grow very slowly between 54-59 degrees F. Between 59-94 degrees F. they develop in a normal manner, growing rapidly and developing chains of cells. When the proper food for them is available, the wall becomes swollen and exhibits the early stages of mother formation. As the temperature rises even higher, they appear as long and thread-like, transparent filaments. The exact temperature to be used will depend on the organism in the process being employed. A temperature of 80 degrees F. to 85 is usually optimum for acetification.

First Make Cider

There are no hard and fast rules or formulas to follow, but the two most important factors to consider are the maturity and variety of the apples to be used in making your cider.

Firm, ripe apples—ripe enough to eat out of your hand—make the best cider and give the highest yield. The best cider is usually made from a blend of different varieties of apples. A blend provides an appealing balance of sweetness, tartness and tang, as well as aromatic overtones. A single variety of apple seldom makes a satisfactory cider. However, a few of the familiar varieties—Gravenstein, Newton-Pippin and McIntosh—have been used alone successfully, but only at the peak of their maturity. A blend of three or more varieties is better. Varieties that have a somewhat neutral juice flavor—such as Rome Beauty—may be used in fairly large proportions because of the ability to pick up and merge the more pronounced flavors of other available varieties.

To make sure you get a premium-quality cider, taste samples of each lot of apples. Also taste samples of trial blends of juices. A good blend should include sweet subacid apples—Baldwin, Hubbardston, Rome Beauty, Stark, Delicious, Grimes and Cortland—grown primarily for eating raw. This group usually is used primarily for most of the cider. The mildly acid to slightly tart group—Winesap, Jonathan, Stayman, Northern Spy, York Imperial, Wealthy, R. I. Greening and Newtown-Pippin—add character to cider. Varieties in the aromatic group–Delicious, Golden Delicious, Winter Banana, Ribston and McIntosh–have outstanding fragrance, aroma and flavor that are carried over into the cider.

Crab apples, in the astringent group, provide tannin–a constituent difficult to obtain in making a high-grade cider. The juices of this astringent group also are highly acidic. Only a small quantity of these apples should be used in the blend. Other astringent apples are: Florence, Hibernal, Red Siberian, Transcendent and Martha.

Extracting the Juice

Always use sound, clean apples. They may be the small sizes, promptly gathered drops, fruits sorted out of the market grade because of mediocre color or finish. They may also be the best you can find. Wash, dry, remove any bruises and core your apples. If you think that the apples have a wax coating on the peels, you might choose to not include the peels in your pulp. Seeds and cores and peels have a high procyanidin content which is a cause of postbottling haze. All equipment must be clean. Reduce your apples to a pulp/mash with whatever means you have chosen: knife, blender or food processor. If you have purchased a cider press which also has an "apple eater" feature, you probably already have apple juice.

Otherwise, to press the pulp, line your pressing container with a clean press cloth (cotton sheeting will do). Have the edges long enough to fold back over the container. Scoop some of the pulp into the container and press it down with your hands. The juice will start to trickle out into your collection container. Fill the container with the pulp to about 3 inches thick, cover the pulp with the excess edges of your cloth. This forms a layer of pulp. Repeat this process 2 or 3 times. So, now you have several layers in press cloth. You will have to use your own judgment how much is right depending upon the type of press you are using. Also, instructions will come with your particular press. Place the pressing board on top and begin to apply pressure in the manner prescribed by your equipment. If it is a homemade cider press, then you would be pressing down with the added aid of bricks and weights. If you bought a standard cider/wine press, you will be turning the handle on a large screw. Apply pressure slowly to avoid rupturing the press cloths. Build up pressure and hold for a while. Work at pressing your juice all day until all the juice has been removed.

There should be several layers of cheesecloth secured over the container which will collect the juice. This is the first filtering of your juice. As soon as the juice is pressed from the apple pulp, strain it again prior to letting it settle for 12 to 36 hours. Make sure the juice is kept at 40 degrees F. or less during this settling process so that fermentation will not start until you are ready for it to start. Be sure your settling container is well covered.

When the settling is completed, draw the juice off, without disturbing the sediment, by using your siphon.

If you are not ready to start the fermentation process, you can keep your cider under refrigeration until you are ready. Cider cooled immediately after pressing and stored at a temperature between 32 degrees and 36 degrees F. retains the original flavor for 1 to 2 weeks without danger of fermentation. Settling can take place under refrigeration. The best method for preserving the fresh flavor of cider is freezing. You can retain your cider and its quality for a least a year. No heat treatment is needed. Freeze the juice as soon after settling as possible. Use containers of glass or plastic and fill them to about 90 percent of capacity to allow for expansion.

Pasteurized cider keeps indefinitely without fermenting. The juice is heated to 170 degrees F. for 10 minutes. Heat the juice in a stainless steel container and then pour the hot cider immediately into clean containers that have been preheated with warm water and cap at once. Place the containers in a tub or sink of warm water. Remove after several minutes and allow them to cool in the air. This method of pasteurizing is satisfactory for batches of 50 gallons or less. A pour spout at the bottom of the heating container is helpful in filling the containers.

Alcoholic Fermentation

You will have already decided at this point what kind of container you will be using for this fermentation process. Discuss this with your supplier, if you have one. Barrels have been used traditionally and are available through a supplier. If you buy a new barrel, be sure to keep it full of water long enough to swell the staves, to prevent leaking. When the barrel is tight and empty, treat the barrel with a solution of soda ash and lye to rid it of strong unpleasant tastes. Thoroughly rinse the barrel until it is 100 percent clean. Remember not to use a barrel which has had vinegar in it for this process because any residue of acetic acid will interfere with the alcoholic fermentation process.

Natural, Unhurried Process

Fill your barrel or 4- to 6-gallon crock two-thirds full of sweet cider. Leave the bung hole in the barrel open but covered with screen or something to keep flies out. Be sure any other type of container also has an opening to allow air. Now, let nature take its course. Fermentation will start in about a day. If there is too much sugar in your juice or the temperature is too high, it will "work" too fast. The process can be slowed down by moving the barrel to a cooler place. If it is working too slowly, no hissing will be heard and no white bubbles will appear. Add some sugar to speed up the fermentation process. You can test how much sugar is in your cider with your hydrometer which gives a specific gravity reading. If the hydrometer reads 1.070 (meaning .07 sugar), the resulting cider will come up to about normal alcoholic content.

Keep the fermenting cider in a cool place, where the temperature is 45 to 50 degrees F. and no more. I would like to point out here that we are talking about the natural, unhurried process of alcoholic fermentation. Leave the "working" alone until the bubbles and hissing of gas have subsided completely.

The minute the process ends, be sure to be there to take the next step. Siphon the fermented cider into clean containers.

Faster Process

Because it takes time for the yeast to work and grow naturally, some people prefer to add a culture of active yeast. Through the addition of wine yeast, S. ellipsoideus, to the cider juice, the yeast quickly gain control over other organisms, and the sugar in the juice is changed into alcohol before any other bacteria have an opportunity to attack it.

It is most important that all the sugar be used up before the acetic bacteria are given their chance, for even a very small amount of acetic acid interferes with the growth of yeast. About 1 yeast cake is needed for every 4 gallons or less of cider juice. If you decided to use yeast, mix 1 yeast cake thoroughly with a little juice and then stir the mixture into the entire batch. Using the yeast, the container should be stored in a place of about 70 degrees F. It must not be covered tightly. Within a few days a violent fermentation will begin. At the end of the fourth day, and each day after that, the mixture should be tested by means of your sugar hydrometer. When the readings remain the same and do not decrease, it means that all the sugar in the juice has been converted into alcohol and the fermentation is complete. Siphon the fermented cider into clean containers.

Racking

This is the process where the fermenting cider is siphoned off into clean containers when the white bubbles appear on the surface. This is a form of filtering, and part of the natural, unhurried, unprocessed process. If you want to take your time, you may also want to rack your cider several times during this fermentation process.

Acetic Acid Fermentation

Your alcoholic cider is now fairly clear and there is no more hissing. You can test the alcohol level with your testing equipment. Use your equipment until you feel confident testing by taste. Fill a clean crock or barrel three-quarters full of the alcohol-fermented juice. The container may be one that has previously contained good vinegar, for now is the time for the Acetobacter bacteria to take over and convert the alcohol to vinegar. Again, this process is a slow one unless it is helped along by the addition of a starter. What better starter could you find than a good vinegar? The vinegar should be unpasteurized. Any good strong vinegar will do, but one containing "mother" is best. Add about one part vinegar to four parts cider. These vinegars are available at any health food store. The home method may take four to six months. When the Acetobacter are allowed to work at their own, unhurried pace, the quality of the product is greatly enhanced. The slow method produces a very heavy, rich, smooth product. Long aging periods also add to the subtle aromas and tastes. The slow process carries with it more risks because it takes more time. The more time there is involved, the more time for things to go wrong.

If you use a crock, cover it with a double layer of cheesecloth to keep out dust and flies. If the crock is kept in a place with

light, put a lid lightly on top to exclude the light but not the air.
At a temperature of about 70 degrees F. the alcohol will be
converted into acetic acid in 4 to 6 months.

After a few days a thin film will appear on the surface of the
fermented cider. This is the "mother of vinegar," and care
should be taken not to disturb this film. Test the vinegar with a
hydrometer and when the hydrometer registers zero in alcoholic
content, the vinegar is ready to move on to the next step.

Aging

While the Acetobacter are still working in the cider vinegar,
it is aged to improve the taste. Aging mellow the vinegar. Some
people think a minimum of six months is need for cider vinegar
to mature completely. The longer it is aged, the more subtle
qualities will appear. Aging should be carried out in a tightly
sealed container that has been filled to the top. Aging is also
important because it gives the cider vinegar a chance to settle
some more which improves the visual quality.

Clarification, Filtering and Fining

These processes are basically to help clear your product.
Clarification of vinegar is primarily for appearance and can be
detrimental to taste and aroma. It is not necessary for the novice
vinegar maker to incur the added expense at this point.

Cider vinegar has a tendency to clear during fermentation. If
you want to filter your vinegar further, you can obtain filtration
kits from your supplier.

An alternative to rough filtration is fining, the process of adding substances that will collect the suspended materials and then settle to the bottom of the container. Fining reduces the total load of suspended material, principally Acetobacter. Good quality bentonite is popular for fining vinegar. It is an inert volcanic ash that imparts little or no taste and is relatively quick acting. Some people like Isinglass which is made from the cleaned, dried bladders of sturgeon or other freshwater fish. Other materials used are gelatin, tannin, potassium ferrocyanide casein and powdered dried blood (Diggs 1989).

Pasteurization

While air is so important during the process of turning alcohol into acetic acid, it is only destructive to vinegar once the process is complete. If you have a large amount of vinegar, you may want to pasteurize it as this is the best method of preserving the flavor and strength. After filtering or fining, pasteurization is used to destroy the active Acetobacter.

Submerge your sealed bottles on a rack or folded towel in a warm-water bath. Heat the water to 140 degrees–160 degrees F. and maintain this temperature for five minutes for pint bottles and ten minutes for quarts.

If you are making small quantities of vinegar, you do not need to pasteurize. Simply bottle in long-neck bottles, cork tightly and seal. Some "mother" may form, but this can be advantageously used when you begin to make another batch of vinegar. Remember, the high heat will destroy beneficial enzymes.

Bottling and Labeling

When aging and all the other processes are finished, you are ready to bottle and label your cider vinegar. The clear vinegar should be siphoned off slowly so that you do not disturb any sedimentation on the bottom or material floating on the top. The bottling should be done all at one time, using every precaution to minimize the vinegar's exposure to air.

In selecting your bottles you want to think about minimizing exposure of your cider vinegar to air. Pint-size bottles with long, thin necks are popular. Make sure to sterilize the bottles before bottling. Corks and wax can be purchased along with your bottles from your supplier. Completely fill each bottle, cork and seal–preferably with wax. Melt your wax in a tall can or other throw-away container in a pan of water. Heat the wax until it is liquid. Before you seal the top, glue a strip of ribbon or string across the top. Dip the top of the bottle into the liquid wax, remove and let dry. You may have to dip the top several times to get a nice solid wax seal. The string or ribbon is to make it easier to break the wax seal when you want to open the bottle.

After you have finished sealing all your bottles, label your cider vinegar. Note the materials used, the quantity made, the acid strength (5 percent), date of production, date of aging and date of bottling.

Storage and Aging

If the bacteria that make acetic acid from alcohol are left exposed to air, they will convert the vinegar to carbon dioxide and water. Now the oxygen is undesirable. The acid level will begin to fall. To prevent this from happening, several things can be done. Pasteurization will kill the active Acetobacter when the temperature is raised, and you can be careful to fill your narrow-necked bottles completely.

You should now store your cider vinegar in a cool place, 49 to 50 degrees F., for at least six months to one year. The longer it is stored, the better it will taste.

Defects and Problems

Some problems encountered in home production of cider vinegar are falling mothers, vinegar flies, vinegar mites and vinegar eels.

Falling Mother of Vinegar

In the slow, home production process the mother sometimes falls. Wash and rinse your hands well before putting them into the vinegar. Make a wooden raft for the mother to float on and with the use of a clean container, remove the mother from the bottom and place it on the raft. Regular aeration may stop mothering–meaning don't shake your containers.

Vinegar flies

These tiny flies find fruit and fruit by-products. They don't eat much. If the larvae of these flies get into your cider vinegar, they can deteriorate the vinegar. Avoid vinegar spills and clean up spills and leaks immediately. If the cider vinegar containers have openings, screen them.

Vinegar mites

Your production space must be very clean. These mites breed rapidly in the right conditions of warmth and moisture; and if they get in the vinegar, they can also spoil it. Hot water or steam will kill them. If the infestation is bad, fumigate with sulphur.

Vinegar eels

A vinegar eel is 1/16 of an inch long and looks like a worm. They somehow find their way into vinegar production. They can be seen by the naked eye when you hold a glass of vinegar up to the light. They are harmless if swallowed but who wants eels swimming in the cider vinegar? Pasteurization and filtration will eliminate the eels.

CHAPTER 7

BRANDS OF CIDER VINEGAR ON THE MARKET

The information presented here is from the product label plus additional information provided by the companies.

My letters of inquiry basically asked the following questions:

1. From what do you make your apple cider vinegar?
2. Do you use whole apples or just peels and cores?
3. Do you add sulfur dioxide?
4. Do you pasteurize?
5. Do you age your cider vinegar? For how long?

BRAND:

INFORMATION:

SPECTRUM NATURALS VINEGAR

Description:

From Certified Organic Apples grown in pesticide free orchards to produce a premier quality vinegar with a delightful flavor and full bouquet.

Ingredients:

Certified organic raw unpasteurized filtered apple cider vinegar. Contains naturally occurring "Mother" of vinegar. 5% acidity.

Nutrition Facts:

Serving Size 1 Tbsp (14 ml.)

Calories: 7

Calories from Fat: 0

Total Fat: 0g

Sodium: 9mg

Total Carbohydrate: 2 g

Sugars: 0g

Total Protein: 0g

Spectrum Naturals Vinegar is made exclusively from organic Gravenstein apples grown in the renown Sonoma County of Northern California. This particular variety of apple produces premier quality vinegar with a delightful flavor and full bouquet.

Like all Spectrum Naturals products, extra care has been taken in bringing this product to the marketplace. Traditionally, vinegar is made from the lowest grade of apples. Spectrum's organic vinegar is made from juice apples, in fact, the same ones used my many well-know organic juice companies.

Unknown to most people, regular apple cider vinegar is often treated with the preservative metabisulfite during fermentation. This treatment is not required to be listed on the label. Spectrum's vinegar is free of this treatment, as well as any other preservatives.

Unlike most commercial vinegars, this unfiltered organic vinegar is neither heat-treated or filtered. It still contain the "Mother," a living mixture of beneficial bacteria and enzymes. Natural sediment occurs in the bottle as molecules of pectin connect in strand-like chains. When this sediment becomes congealed, it can be broken up simply by shaking before use.

Spectrum does have a filtered cider vinegar product, and it is filtered with diatomaceous or fullers earth as a filter mechanism.

The vinegar is matured depending on temperature, microbial activity and quality of the apple juice from 30 to 90 days.

*   *   *

BRAND: SOLANA GOLD ORGANIC VINEGAR

INFORMATION: Description:

Vinegar is fundamental. It's universal like water. Cook, clean, bathe and nourish with it, like people did in simpler times. Apple cider vinegar can also lessen the harmful effects of food bacteria like E. Coli, concluded a 1996 joint research study at Nagoya Medical University in Japan.

See the veil floating in your vinegar? That's called The Mother, and is unique to apple cider vinegar. As raw apple juice is fermented to hard cider, protein enzymes link into a floating, molecular chain. Many manufactures unnecessarily expose vinegar to clarifying agents, heat and filtration. Looks 'advertising pretty', but what happened to the beneficial dormant living-enzyme proteins?

Solana Gold apples are grown without the use of synthetic fertilizers, herbicides or pesticides.
- USDA Organic
- KSA Kosher
- Raw & Unfiltered
- Made with the Veil of the Mother
Ingredients:
Organic raw apple cider vinegar and water to 5% acidity (unfiltered, unpasteurized).
Nutrition Facts:
Serving Size: 1 Tbsp
Calories: 5
All the same as Spectrum.

BRAND: <u>BRAGG LIVE FOOD PRODUCTS VINEGAR</u>

INFORMATION: <u>Description:</u>

Delicious, ideal pick-me-up at home, work, sports or gym. Perfect taken 3 times daily—upon arising, mid-morning and mid-afternoon–1 to 2 tsp Bragg Organic Vinegar in 8 oz. glass of purified water and (optional 1 to 2 tsp organic honey, 100% Maple syrup, Blackstrap molasses or 4 drops Stevia).

Contains the amazing Mother of Vinegar which occurs naturally as strand-like chains of connected protein molecules. If sediment occurs, shake before using.

<u>Ingredients:</u>
Certified Bragg organic raw apple cider vinegar is unfiltered, unheated, unpasteurized and 5% acidity.

<u>Nutrition Facts:</u>
Same as Spectrum.

*   *   *

BRAND: EDEN FOODS VINEGAR

INFORMATION: Description:

The finest organically grown apples are naturally fermented with 'mother' of vinegar, a quality indicator appearing as cloudiness in the final product. Raw and unpasteurized, patiently aged in cedar wood vats. A traditional health food used for centuries in hundreds of ways.

Ingredients:

Organic apple cider vinegar diluted with water to 5% acidity.

Nutrition Facts:

Same as Spectrum.

CHAPTER 8

ANSWERS TO QUESTIONS

The following is a summary of answers to questions concerning apple cider vinegar.

What is apple cider vinegar?

Apple cider vinegar is a vinegar, acetic acid, made from apples, apple peels and apple cores.

Why does it work?

The answers to this question are varied depending upon whether you are talking about medicinal uses, cleaning uses or the preserving of foods. In brief, why it works for medicinal purposes are: It is principally acetic acid and lethal to many microorganisms; it can help maintain the acid-alkaline balance of the body; and it is a good source of potassium which is essential to the body. Why it works for cleaning purposes has much to do with it being a mild acid. Why it works for preserving food has to do with the bactericidal properties of acetic acid.

How is it made?

Apples are cleaned, dried, reduced to a pulp and the juice pressed out of the pulp. The juice is put in containers for the sugar in the juice to ferment into alcohol by natural yeast. The alcoholic cider is then put into clean containers and allowed to ferment into acetic acid by Acetobacter bacteria. It is aged, filtered, pasteurized (generally), bottled and stored.

What is good quality cider vinegar?

A good quality cider vinegar is one made from organic whole apples, using as little as possible of the peels and cores. It is made in an unhurried manner which would allow sediments to settle out. It is aged adequately and has as few additives as possible. If you want the enzymes, you would not want it pasteurized.

Why are additives added?

They are added to stabilize the vinegar and for clarification. Most buyers prefer a clear, bright vinegar. Preservatives retard the growth of spoilage organisms.

What additives are added?

In most production plants, the cider stock is fortified with nutrients before acetification, i.e. ammonium carbonate, ammonium sulfate and ammonium monophosphate..

If a cider vinegar is not well-aged, it may be treated with activated carbon or with Polyclar AT after rough filtration. This is done to absorb and remove the polyphenols which cause postbottling haze.

Various agents have been added to cider vinegar at the bottling stage, mostly to prevent excessive haze formation. The most effective is sulfur dioxide. Ascorbic acid is sometimes added but considered less effective in haze reduction. Pectin and gum arabic have also been added to stabilize vinegar against haze formation.

Why is sulfur dioxide used in the production of vinegar?

Preservatives retard the growth of most spoilage organisms, but they may not stop growth completely. Beech (1958) reported that the addition of sulfur dioxi de to apple juice reduced the bacterial population to almost nothing. This was the result of the addition of 150 ppm sulfur dioxide. The surviving yeasts were primarily fermenting types. Sulfur dioxide encouraged selection of a fermentative yeast flora. Sulfur dioxide is added to apple juice based on the pH and is in the form of a sodium metabisulfite solution. The legal limit in the United States is 200 ppm sulfur dioxide.

The juice/sulphur mixture is allowed to stand for 24 hours and then it is put into clean sterile vessels for fermentation and fermenting yeast cultures are added.

The sulphur dioxide in the juice must be removed. It is done by aerating the mixture and adding food-grade hydrogen peroxide. The finished product is inspected for any trace of sulphur dioxide because of allergic sensitivity to it. Strict laws are in force on the use of sulphur products.

Sulfur dioxide is also added to prevent excessive haze formation. It has been found to be the most effective agent for this purpose. Its effectiveness arises because of its antimicrobial properties, which are enhanced by the low pH, and from its antioxidant, enzyme-inhibiting and carbonyl-binding functions, which effectively block all polyphenol polymerization.

Some of the benefits of using sulphur dioxide sterilized fruit juice are 1) sugars ferment almost completely, 2) undesirable yeasts and lactic acid bacteria are dead, 3) the vinegar clears quicker and 4) acetification proceeds more rapidly.

What are some of the side effects of sulfur dioxide?
It destroys vitamin B1 and can cause severe reactions in asthmatics. The particular group at risk appears to be 5-10 percent of asthmatics (Simon et al. 1982). It is important to include sulfite on ingredient labels to alert sensitive individuals. The general public should not have an adverse reaction to sulfite when used at recommended levels. This additive has caused at least seven deaths according to the New York Library Desk Reference (1989 ed.), "Chemical Additives." This reference further states, "This additive is unsafe in the amounts normally consumed or is poorly tested." They suggest it be avoided. They do not specify what they mean by "amounts normally consumed."

Do you need to include additives when you make your own?

Kits with instructions are available through your equipment supplier. For your home production product adding sulfur dioxide is unnecessary as long as you make certain that your work area is kept exceptionally clean and you use good quality apples with no bruises or rotten spots. No, you do not need to include additives.

What is Patulin?

Patulin is a fungal toxin that may be present in apple products. It inhibits the growth of a number of bacteria, yeasts and molds. In a study by Lindroth (1980) little intact patulin is absorbed from the gastrointestinal tract. The toxic effects are caused by unidentified derivatives of patulin breakdown.

Patulin contamination of apple products can be easily controlled by using only sound fruit. Fruit may be trimmed to remove patulin that is concentrated in damaged portions of the tissue. Potassium sorbate and sodium proprionate inhibit patulin growth. Sulfur dioxide, potassium sorbate and sodium benzoate retard patulin production in apple juice. The toxin can be physically removed by treatment with activated charcoal. Patulin is reduced by fermenting yeasts. Production of fermented cider is a means of reclaiming contaminated apple juice.

Oral administration of patulin causes stomach irritation, nausea and vomiting in humans. It is carcinogenic when injected. However, carcinogenicity has not been demonstrated when it is taken orally.

Why is apple cider vinegar generally pasteurized?

Cider vinegar is pasteurized to kill living organisms in the product, i.e. Acetobacter bacteria or vinegar eels. It helps to stabilize the product.

How does pasteurization affect the quality?

It does stabilize the product but it also destroys beneficial enzymes.

Do you need to pasteurize when you make your own?

No, but you may want to if you are making large quantities in order to stabilize your vinegar.

How does using cores and peels affect the product?

Cores and peels contain more procyanidins than the rest of the apple. Procyanidins are the major producer of polyphenolic haze. So, the more cores and peels you use, the more postbottling haze problems you will have.

Can apple cider vinegar adversely affect you?

There is no record of cider vinegar adversely affecting anyone. However, good judgment should be used and the quality of the cider vinegar you are using should be taken into consideration.

GLOSSARY

Acetobacter—The bacteria in vinegar that cause the conversion of alcohol to acetic acid.

Acetification—The technical name for the process of converting alcohol to acetic acid by Acetobacter.

Acid-Alkaline Balance—The balance of acid and alkaline reactions in the body's system, i.e. urine should normally be on the acid side and blood on a slightly alkaline side.

Clarification—The filtering of vinegar to clarify it so that it will be clear and bright. The vinegar may be treated with activated carbon or with Polyclar AT after rough filtration to absorb and remove polyphenols which are responsible for postbottle hazes.

Fermentation—The conversion of sugar to alcohol and carbon dioxide by yeast and the conversion of alcohol to acetic acid by Acetobacter.

Fining—The process of adding substances to cider vinegar that will collect the suspended materials and then settle to the bottom of the container. Fining reduces the amount of suspended material, principally Acetobacter, and may help to reduce the haze contributing polyphenols.

Maturation—After the acetification process, the vinegar is pumped into tanks for storage and maturation. Maturation is an important step in the process because it helps in the clarification and development of the flavor.

Mother of Vinegar (Acetobacter xylinum)—The vinegar-generating organisms which secrete sheets of cellulose. It is used as a starter for fresh batches of cider to start the acetification process.

Pasteurization—The temperature of the cider vinegar is raised to 140-160 degrees F. which destroys the active Acetobacter. The high heat will destroy beneficial enzymes also.

Procyanidins—One of the four major classes of polyphenols in apples and the one most responsible for postbottling haze.

Racking—During the first fermentation process of converting apple juice into apple cider, the cider is drawn off and put into clean casks several times. It is also a form of filtering as sediment settles to the bottom. As soon as white bubbles appear, it is time to rack again. This was one step in the early method of making alcoholic cider.

Ultrafiltration—An alternative method of stabilizing cider vinegar. Raw vinegar is pumped continuously past membranes with typical cutoff of 50,000 molecular weight. It is also partly recirculated. It helps remove acetification debris and Acetobacters.

Vinegar eels—Vinegar eels, nematodes of the species Anguillula aceti, are carried by fruit flies. They live at the top of fermentation and storage vessels, independent of light and oxygen. They may appear at any stage in the production of vinegar.

Vinegar mites—Not as much of a problem as eels, but breed rapidly in the right conditions of warmth and moisture.

BIBLIOGRAPHY/REFERENCES

Beech, "The Yeast Flora of Apple Juice and Ciders," J. Appl. Bacterial, 21: 257–66, 1958.

Birdsong, Craig, "Household Cleaning Recipes," Service in Action, CSUCE, No. 9.502, 8/88.

Bragg, Paul C. and Patricia Bragg, "Apple Cider Vinegar Health System." Health Science, Santa Barbara, CA, 1989.

Bricklin, Mark, "Rodale's Encyclopedia of Natural Home Remedies." Rodale Press, Inc. 1982.

Buchman, D. D., "Herbal Medicine–The Natural Way to Get Well and Stay Well." Gramercy Publishing Co., NY, 1980.

"Chemical Additives," The New York Public Library Desk Reference (1989 ed.), Simon & Schuster, Inc. NY, 523.

"Country Lore—Bricks Fix," Mother Earth News, No. 97 (Jan/Feb 1986), 36.

Crawford, Mildred A., "Stain Removal from Fabrics," Service in Action, CSUCE, No 8.500, 1/88.

Diggs, Lawrence J., "Vinegar—The User Friendly Standard Text, Reference and Guide to Appreciating, Making and

Enjoying Vinegar." Quiet Storm Trading Company, Sf, CA, 1989.

Hanssen, Maurice, "Cider Vinegar." Arco Publishing Co., Inc., NY, 1978.

Harris, Ben Charles, "Kitchen Medicines." Weathervane Books, NY, 1968.

"Hints on Cider and Cider Vinegar," Colorado State University Cooperative Extension Service, LA 9276, 1975.

Jarvis, D. C., M.D., "Folk Medicine—A Vermont Doctor's Guide to Good Health." Fawcett Publishing, Greenwich, Conn., 1958.

Kahn, J. H., G. B. Nickel, and H. A. Conner, "Identification of Volatile Components in Vinegars by GLC-MS," J. Agric Food Chem, 20: 214–18, 1972.

Kendall, Pat, Ph.D., R. D., "Food Preservation Without Sugar or Salt," Service in Action, CSUCE, No. 9.302, 7/88.

Kendall, Pat, Ph.D., R. D., and Carol Schultz, M. S., C.H.E., "Making Pickles at Home," Service in Action, CSUCE, No. 9.304, 12/89.

Lea, Andrew G. H., "Processed Apple Products." Van Nostrand Reinhold, NY, 1989.

Lindroth, S., "Occurrence, Formation and Detoxification of Patulin Mycotoxin." Material Processing Technol Publ. 24, Technical Research Center, Espoo, Finland, 1980.

Malstrom, Stan D, N. D., M. T., "Own Your Own Body." Keats Publishing, Inc., New Canaan, Conn., 1977.

Orton, Vrest, "The American Cider Book." Farrar, Straus and Giroux, NY, 1973.

Rinzler, Carol Ann, "The Complete Book of Herbs, Spices and Condiments." Henry Holt and Company, NY, 1990.

Rose, Jeanne, "Herbs and Things." Workman Publishing Company, NY, 1972.

Scott, Cyril, "Cider Vinegar–Nature's Great Health Promoter and Safest Treatment of Obesity." Thorson Publishing Group, Bungay, Suffolk, 1982.

"Senior Counselor," Special 1991 Edition, 26-27.

Seranne, Ann, "The Complete Book of Home Preserving." Doubleday & Company, Inc., NY, 1953.

Shuttleworth, John, "The Mother Earth News Almanac." Bantam Books, NY, 1973.

Simon, R. A., L. Green, and D. D. Stevenson, "The Incidence of Ingested Metabisulfite Sensitivity in an Asthmatic Population," J. Allergy Clin. Immunol., 69:118, 1982.

Smock, R .M., and A .M. Neubert, "Apples and Apple Products." Interscience Publishers, NY, 1950.

Thesen, Karen, "Country Remedies from Pantry, Field and Garden." Harper & Row, 1979.

"Vagabond Vinegar," FDA Consumer, Vol 22, June 88, 32.

Vaughn, Reese H., "Vinegar," The Encyclopedia Americana (1980 ed.) Vol 28, 134.

"Vinegar," The New Encyclopedia Britannica (1988 ed.) XII, 380.

978-0-595-41237-2
0-595-41237-8

Made in the USA
Middletown, DE
26 December 2017